Praise for *One Got Past...*

'What a great read! Great advice and very true.'
Joel 'Parko' Parkinson, three times winner of the Hawaiian Triple Crown of Surfing and father of three

'I've never been a big fan of soccer, or the people who play it, really. That all quickly changed upon reading One Got Past the Keeper; *a tremendous story of mateship, relationships and parenting. A must read for any man who is a dad, has a dad, is about to become a dad or who thinks they one day might be a dad.'*
Steve Le Marquand, actor (*Underbelly, Beneath Hill 60, Last Train to Freo*) and recent father

'This is just the sort of information new fathers need – stories of mateship and being blokes together that many men will recognise.'
Dr Richard Fletcher, author of *The Dad Factor*, leader of the Fathers and Families Research Program at the University of Newcastle and experienced father

'Even after having two kids and being step mamma to three more, One Got Past the Keeper *offered vital insights I didn't even realise I'd been missing. Every woman entertaining ideas about breeding should read this book, it really opens up a world of compassion (and humour!) often difficult to find for our fellas during that incredible but challenging transition into parenthood. One of the easiest to devour and giving books I've read in a very long time.'*
Mel Bampton, ex-triple J presenter and music and books editor, *yen* magazine, and mother

ONE GOT PAST THE KEEPER

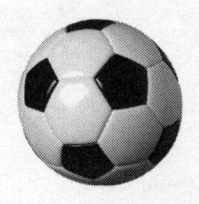

WRITTEN BY NEIL YOUNG, JIM ROBERTS, YARI MCGAULEY, ROSS DEVINE, RICK FITZGERALD AND NICK FOLEY

hachette
AUSTRALIA

Note to readers: This is a rare book about fatherhood in that it was not written by anyone who knew what they were talking about until they became a parent. None of the men involved has any relevant qualifications or is an expert in any associated field (including the football field). Although every effort has been made to give you the best information, we are merely men – new dads not doctors, fresh pappas not professional footballers, and so anything we say about fatherhood or football (or anything else really) should be treated with very little reverence and maybe even slight disdain.

hachette
AUSTRALIA

Published in Australia and New Zealand in 2011
by Hachette Australia
(an imprint of Hachette Australia Pty Limited)
Level 17, 207 Kent Street, Sydney NSW 2000
www.hachette.com.au

10 9 8 7 6 5 4 3 2 1

Copyright © Neil Young, Jim Roberts, Yari McGauley, Ross Devine, Rick Fitzgerald, Nick Foley 2011

This book is copyright. Apart from any fair dealing for the purposes of private study, research, criticism or review permitted under the *Copyright Act 1968*, no part may be stored or reproduced by any process without prior written permission. Enquiries should be made to the publisher.

National Library of Australia
Cataloguing-in-Publication data

National Library of Australia Cataloguing-in-Publication entry:
Fertile FC (Soccer team)
One got past the keeper / Fertile FC.

ISBN 978 0 7336 2791 0 (pbk.)

Fertile FC (Soccer team)
Fatherhood – Anecdotes.
Parenting – Anecdotes.
Soccer teams – Anecdotes.

306.8742

Cover design by Christabella Designs
Cover photograph courtesy of Sally James
Text design by Christabella Designs
Typeset in Sabon by Kirby Jones
Printed in Australia by Griffin Press, Adelaide, an Accredited ISO AS/NZS 4001:2004 Environmental Management Systems printer

The paper this book is printed on is certified against the Forest Stewardship Council® Standards. Griffin Press holds FSC chain of custody certification SGS-COC-005088. FSC promotes environmentally responsible, socially beneficial and economically viable management of the world's forests.

Dedicated to Antonio

CONTENTS

BEFORE KICK-OFF — ix

SEASON ONE — 1
The Rusty Trombones FC — 3

SEASON TWO — 25
Fertile FC — 27
Jim's story — 41
Yari's story — 73
Ross' story — 107
Rick's story — 153
Neil's story — 185
Antonio's story — 221

SEASON THREE — 225
The Trombones FC — 227

EXTRA TIME — 251
Nick's story — 253

Suggested further reading — 265

'Fatherhood is like a goal-saving tackle. You slide into it and you know it's going to hurt a bit, but you go in anyway. You do it for the team and you give it one hundred per cent commitment. You stay brave, play fair and deal with what happens. And you'd do it again and again for your team.'

A Fertile FC football player who became a father

BEFORE KICK-OFF

WHAT YOU'RE HOLDING RIGHT NOW IS A BOOK WRITTEN BY MEN, primarily for men, particularly those who are about to become fathers. But ladies, if you're reading this, don't put it down just yet – hopefully there's something in here for you as well.

This is the true story of us, six blokes who put together a six-a-side social soccer team, and how we became mates. Initially it was more about the social than the soccer, but united in a desire not to come last, we soon found ourselves united in something much bigger. Whether it was planned, unplanned, or due to the testosterone boost we got playing competitive sport for the first time in years, all of our wives or girlfriends, bar one, became pregnant after our first season together. The question was, no matter how tall, short, fast, slow, macho or sensitive we were – or however good or bad we were at football – did we have what it takes to be good fathers?

Our stories are as different as we are; we all come from different places and different walks of life, but our individual journeys saw us all living within ten kilometres of each other in Northern New South Wales and answering a call to join an amateur football team. Our relationships took different forms: there were fathers in their twenties and fathers in their forties. There were first-time fathers, a 48-year-old first-time father, a father having his second child, a father with a step-child, and a father already with children to a different partner. There were miscarriages, home births, hospital births, a home birth that ended up in hospital, water births, natural births, breech births, an elective caesarean, an emergency caesarean and a lot of morning sickness.

It was from these diverse experiences and backgrounds that this book was 'conceived'. By sharing our team's experiences we hope we have created the book all of us needed as we prepared for fatherhood. Not men's birth stories of standing in the corner of a hospital delivery room watching our loved ones going through it, but going through it ourselves. Complete journeys into fatherhood as we transformed from someone's son into someone's father.

This book explores what the whole experience is like from the man's perspective – from thinking about conception (or not thinking about it for that matter) through each stage of pregnancy, to holding a newborn baby and taking him or her home. We have attempted to openly and honestly share what we felt and experienced as we learned how to become good team players in a completely new team. There are no experts involved here, just real stories told by real men.

SEASON ONE

The Rusty Trombones FC

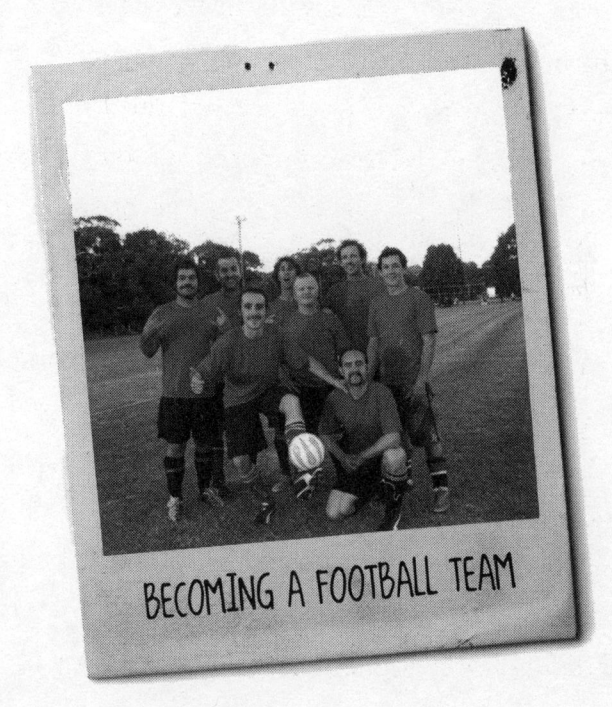

BECOMING A FOOTBALL TEAM

THE RUSTY TROMBONES FC

JIM WAS THE CAPTAIN. HE HAD A FOOTBALL. HE ALSO HAD A vacant block of land next door to the share house where he lived. Jim knew each of us – different men of different ages from different parts of his life. He also knew we were each interested, to varying degrees, in football (or at least sport) and might consider training together and eventually registering a team to enter a local six-a-side soccer comp – more for fun than anything else.

He sent around a group email.

> Are you guys (and friends) interested in being part of the Mullum Maulers (open to suggestions on names) six-a-side soccer team? The season starts in late September I think. The cost is about $60 (plus if we want our own shirts it will be an extra $7). So far I have myself (probably goalie) and Marcello (striker). I reckon we need about eight to ten lads

just in case people can't make it. It is on a Thursday night. Kick-off times change from between 6 p.m. and 8 p.m. It is at Bangalow and beers after the game are mandatory. The game goes for about twenty to twenty-five mins each way. The pitch is half-size and the goals are half-size. There are some good teams, but there will be teams of our standard too (i.e. very average). I need a firm commitment, so if you say yes then you are in! *Jim.*

Although he'd probably say he wasn't a natural leader, Jim took quite naturally to the duties of captain, once he started. We all trusted his ingenuity immediately when – at our first training session – he brilliantly suggested that we park our cars at either end of the vacant block with their headlights on full-beam, so that we could see the ball after the sun went down. We politely applauded his problem-solving abilities, despite the fact that it was extremely challenging running into the full-beam of headlights and trying to take a shot at goal with our eyes closed and not smash a windscreen.

Even though it was unknown to each of us, I think we were all in agreement that one of the reasons for joining a group of men that we didn't really know, to play a sport some of us didn't really understand, was because we could all do with getting a bit fitter. Another reason was that we knew Jim – he was a nice bloke and he'd asked us. Even before we had met, I think we had all individually decided that chasing a ball around a paddock with a bunch of new mates would be more fun than jogging the streets alone at night in an old tracksuit, or swimming laps of the pool on the weekend in baggy budgie smugglers. Fitness and fun – that's what it was all about at this stage of our lives – football would keep us fit, and we'd have some fun doing it.

We had each settled in Northern New South Wales around Byron Bay, a laid-back, lush part of Australia that had been known as a meeting place for thousands of years to the Aboriginal people who came to the area to swap stories, find marriage partners and trade goods with the local Bundjalung people. The close proximity of mountainous volcanic hinterland to the world-class sandbank surfbreaks meant there were often weird weather patterns, including electrical storms and rainbows. This also meant there were some crazy people drawn to the area – the lost and lonely as well as the rich and successful – which all lent to the magic and lore of the place.

Byron Bay was very different from the country towns that surrounded it – it was like a little cosmopolitan tart plonked in the middle of a plate of Aussie meat pies. In Byron Bay you could get a good curry, a great cappuccino and then tandem-skydive to a snorkelling adventure – it was well on the beaten track of every visiting backpacker. But then twenty kilometres in any direction you went back twenty years in time to the quintessential Chinese restaurant and counter meals of rural Australia, with its main street and market, its local radio station and magnificent natural beauty.

At the time of that first training session, some of us hadn't played sport since school and some of us hadn't ever kicked a round ball in our lives. But one thing we all had in common was that we didn't do as much exercise as we did when we were younger. We worked a bit too much and we had comfortable lives – warm dinners and cold beers every night – and the bodies to prove it. But as well as contributing to our new, healthier lifestyles, a team game like football seemed like a good chance to spend time in the company of men and share a cleansing ale or two after some worthy physical exertion, and an opportunity to make like-minded friends locally. A team game such as football would be good for mateship, unless we took it too seriously or didn't take it seriously enough – depending on everyone's differing expectations.

When you stand around in shorts, in a circle of men who you don't know very well, you do your best to make each other feel at ease. Everyone else is doing exactly the same thing, so it's usually an uncomplicated environment of easy chat, easy smiles and easy laughs. The most difficult thing was controlling the football between us.

But eagerness is often more valuable than skill, and that we had in abundance. We also had Jim. Jim was thirty-four, and your typical Aussie surfer–skater. But he also knew a lot about the training tactics used by Sir Alex Ferguson, the most successful manager of Manchester United FC (Football Club) in the English Premier League. Although Jim had lived in Australia most of his adult life, and in the Byron area for five years, he was brought up in Manchester, England, and like most people who came from there, he lived and breathed football. Jim looked like a natural footballer, wiry in an athletic, non-weedy way. He told us he used to play football during every school break and every lunchtime, and then after school he and his mates would head to the park, put down a couple of jumpers for goals and continue playing until the light faded.

Twenty-five years later, as the light faded on another warm spring evening in Northern New South Wales, Jim was joined on the vacant quarter-acre block by Ezza – soon to be known as 'Twinkle-toes' – an old mate of Jim's from Sydney who was in the area for a short time working on the Splendour in the Grass music festival in nearby Byron Bay. He had never kicked a round ball before. A little later, 'Pirate' Steve joined Jim and Ezza. Pirate Steve was a local friend of Jim's who was building a boat to sail away from the impending collapse of the free market economy (he correctly predicted the GFC). He was another who had never played soccer before, and later in the season we could identify which games he had played in because other players always got injured. Also present early that evening was Marcello, an Italian barista from a local café some of us frequented. Marcello was a freestyle football juggler – he had the football moves, and also the disco moves. He was beginning to overstay his Australian visa because 'the garls are sooo bewtiful in Australia'.

I was next to turn up. 'G'day Neil, ready to pull the boots on again?' said Jim as I arrived (with no boots). I had met Jim through our mutual involvement in Uncle – a local mentoring and activities program for boys with absent fathers (although neither Jim nor I were fathers, or considering fatherhood). I was an actor in my late forties and at that point I was definitely looking more portly than sporty. The others told me later that I looked like a cross between a cockney gangster and an eccentric hippy: sarongs, chenille and thongs on a rough, chunky body. I was originally from England and knew how to play football: one, from memories of my childhood; and two, from watching way too much English Premier League on pay TV in the middle of the night in Australia. As the season progressed, I was to become known as 'Rock Solid' because my defensive style of play was somewhat similar to a brick wall.

Rick was next to turn up, he was an ex-builder, ex-fireman and ex-bass player in an eighties rock band. Currently, he was a vegetarian surfer who ran a marketing business. Rick had a deceptive physical appearance: his large head and slouching posture meant he was taller than he looked. He was very Australian; he held court well and was not shy to tell a yarn or two, which were always worth listening to, however long. Rick was originally from the Northern

Beaches of Sydney, he was the new boyfriend of an old friend of Jim's from Sydney. Several years before, Rick had played in the six-a-side soccer comp we planned to enter, so he was our 'inside man'. Jim called him 'Mr Bangalow' because he knew everyone in town. Later, Jim also called him 'Reckless Rick' because of some of his tackles.

The last to arrive was Ross, who'd come straight from his work in Community Development an hour or more away on the Gold Coast. Ross had met Jim through their mutual interest in skateboarding. Ross or 'Happy Hands' – due to his habit of waving his arms around while talking to help you understand his broad Glaswegian accent – had his long dark hair drawn back into a ponytail, which made him look even more Scottish in the most *Braveheart* of ways. He drove a kombi, and was like a hippy in a suit. Ross and his wife hadn't been in the area long and didn't know many people locally, although his endearing ways would soon ensure otherwise. He obviously knew what to do with a football but, equally obviously, he hadn't had the chance to do so for some time.

The seven of us shook hands, grinning, and then tentatively began giggling at each others' lack of ability and coordination when trying to control a football. None of us had football boots. I was wearing steel-capped Blundstones and no one wanted to get in the way of one of my swinging legs. Rick was wearing standard runners and when he moved too fast in one direction he ended up sliding into the fence or bushes of the perimeter. Ross was wearing fashionable but useless fat, unlaced skate shoes. Jim and particularly Marcello were football freaks to the rest of us: they could kick the ball where they wanted it to go, and it went there, regardless of their footwear. While Ezza and Steve, on the other hand, were more likely to take you out with a rugby tackle than fancy footwork. And at some stage during the noisy entertainment, a couple of local barefoot kids we knew joined in and showed us a few tricks.

Thirty minutes later, we were all sitting around on Jim's deck, red-faced and panting. The air was full of the sounds of a typical spring evening in rural Australia: cicadas and beer cans phizting open. There were some strong personalities among the group but no one dominated with too much confidence. Everyone was given space and time as we got to know each other, sharing self-deprecating stories and making each other laugh over a couple of cold ones. We were different ages (more than twenty years between me and the youngest) and some of us had come from the other side of the world to be on that deck on that evening. It was clear that some of us could play football, and some of us couldn't. Some of us could tell a good story, and some of us could listen and laugh – but we were all equally important to the team. Certainly the men among us were not the blokes best at football but maybe the best of blokes.

We discussed a name for our new team, but for some peculiar reason most of the names we came up with had homosexual connotations – like 'Boys United' (instead of Man United), or 'Men in Shorts'. Eventually we went with Ezza and Steve's suggestion of the 'Rusty Trombones FC' – we were indeed rusty. Later we were both amazed and appalled to find out that a 'rusty trombone' is also the name of a rather perverse sexual act. For those amazed, it appealed to our masculine dressing-room sense of impropriety, irresponsibility and indecency, and for those appalled it remained an enduring embarrassment. For Ezza and Pirate Steve it was the funniest thing in the world.

We talked about our new team like a new family, but knew that during the coming six-a-side football comp season – if we managed to get it together to enter – some of us would occasionally be unavailable due to work obligations, social commitments, spontaneous interstate trips or injury. We needed more players to cover, otherwise, with only enough players to fill the team and no substitutes, we'd all be running up and down for the whole of the game until we got giddy and fell over. We knew we had to choose new recruits carefully because anyone who didn't fit our team ethos of 'fitness and fun' probably wouldn't fit in, and definitely wouldn't have fun. For that matter, anyone who wanted to look proficient on a football field, win football matches and *not* have to apologise to his girlfriend or wife the next day for coming home really late in a real state, need not apply. So, just before the deadline of registering new players, we were pleased to welcome Nick, or 'Bootsy', to our ranks.

Nick, originally from the Gold Coast, was an old friend of Jim's new partner. Nick was into surfing and liked to go out and have a good time, but also, somewhat ironically for him, studied naturopathy. He wore an old pair of leather ankle-high boots that reminded us of 'Billy's Boots': an old comic strip in which Billy's boots possessed the magical abilities of their original owner, Jimmy 'Dead-shot' Keen, which turned Billy into a fantastic football player whenever he played in them. Nick's boots fitted, he fitted in well with all of us, but (sadly) his boots weren't really magic.

We had one practice game before the six-a-side comp started proper. Jim had arranged a game against a local high-school team. As we crossed the sports field that evening, our opponents were bobbing and weaving, and heading and passing to each other with the confidence and bravado of youth. We were a bit concerned that they were going to run rings around us until we fell into a panting pile, but it was during that game that we discovered one of our core strengths. What we lacked in fitness, speed, agility, skill, stamina and talent we could make up for with a mixture of enthusiasm, determination and possibly even intimidation. There are few things more unsettling to a teenage boy than the unpredictability of an uncoordinated older man rushing towards him as he comes to terms with the inevitability of middle age. We won comfortably thanks mainly to Marcello. Marcello was a really good football player and could beat several defenders before scoring, but I couldn't help thinking that it might be more fun to lose and get the ball passed to me occasionally.

Two weeks later we came to the Bangalow Sporting Fields for the first time, and we were all a little impressed and a little overwhelmed. We could see the floodlights in the distance as we drove in. There were eight illuminated football pitches, each with a crowd of supporters and friends around it watching the games, and with another two teams getting ready to go on next. It was hard to park and there was nowhere to change or shower, but there was a toilet block, a sausage sizzle and a canteen selling beers and softies – all that was needed. We felt a collective rush of excitement as we entered the throng of activity with our kit bags over our shoulders and our bodies as ready as they would ever be to play competitive football.

The Bangalow Summer Sixes competition had started a few years before as an October to December, ten-week kick-around in the soccer off-season when some of the players from the Bangalow team divided themselves into smaller six-a-side teams. An urban (or should that be rural) myth exists that for the first season they backed a HiAce van up to the oval, opened the backdoors, and each week a different team would be drawn to choose the music that would be played at full volume over the fields.

The rules were pretty simple. Six-a-side football teams with up to four subs allowed to interchange, playing on a half-size soccer pitch using half-size goals that made a lovely tinny 'crack!' when you scored. Twenty-five minutes each half, no offside and a unwritten code of no stupid, dangerous tackles. It cost $550 to enter a team – that worked out at about $60 a player for seven games and then a final series in which you could win a trophy if you won a quarter-final, a semi-final and then a grand final. There were around fifty teams registered (about two-thirds men, one-third women) that played at 6 p.m., 7 p.m. or 8 p.m. on eight pitches under floodlights with real refs who could give you a yellow card or a red card or suspend you for foul play.

As we chucked our bags down and began to get changed, it was pretty obvious to anyone watching that we hadn't played before, or at least not for a few years. Many of the other squads of young men looked to be out-of-season A or B grade players out to keep fit – some had sponsorship endorsements on their shirts and some were young enough to be my son. Thankfully, there were also a few other scruffy looking groups. While all the fit young things stretched, warmed-up and juggled footballs between them, we unwrapped our brand-new 'bargain bin' boots and compared notes on prices paid in op-shops for socks and shorts. Wisely, a couple of paperback books were on hand for those who didn't have the necessary shin-pads needed in order to comply with regulations. And, to complete our kit, Jim handed out a simple red T-shirt to each player, the same colour as the Manchester United jersey and, as Jim pointed out, the same colour worn by such great players as George

Best, Dennis Law and Bobby Charlton. We all smiled and nodded and gave Jim seven bucks for T-shirts that still had the folds in them, had a large black number on the back, and were bloody hot to play in.

Before this first game, the anticipation was huge. We were to play the Chefs, not surprisingly a team made up of local chefs, cooks and kitchen hands. Once changed, we all walked on to the field and began shooting some balls at the goal and trying to get a corner kick across for someone's head to meet the incoming ball. Not overly impressively. The Chefs were warming up at the other end of the pitch and it looked as if they hadn't played a lot before either. They were wearing cut-off chequered chef's pants, their numbers were drawn on with permanent marker and it wouldn't be too harsh to say their pasta probably far surpassed their passing. We were relieved to see another team who were playing with the same ethos as us – 'kick and giggle'.

Jim called us together before the kick-off to explain our positions and what was expected of us. Marcello would play up front, Jim and Ross would start in midfield, I was at centre back because although I was short, I had a loud voice and was tough in the tackle, and Rick (also tough in the tackle) would partner me at the back. Nick was in goal and Ezza and Pirate Steve were substitutes. Steve didn't have boots, so every time he came on, he had to swap with the player coming off – the quicker we tried to swap boots, the longer it took, but the funnier it was. Even though it was a well-matched game of good intentions – with Marcello taking his dribbling and shooting far too seriously – rather embarrassingly, we won 9–1! We only had expectations of losing, so to win so emphatically was unbelievable and put everyone on a high. We all shared handshakes, backslaps and beers with each other and our worthy opponents – football was the real winner that evening, that and the bloke who sold beers at the canteen.

Our second game was against the Bangalow Bullfrogs – our first game against a football team of players who played football. Marcello didn't show up because he had played with some of the other team before – a reason the rest of us found hard to understand. Jim's coaching tip was 'Five people behind the ball at all times – and don't cry.' We lost 2–1. For us, the game was a triumph, mainly because we managed not to get thrashed. The other team's average age was about twenty-three, and none of them was wearing airport novels, thongs or cardboard from the case of beer we'd just bought as shin-pads in their socks. Jim started to show his competitive spirit and almost had a fight with a bloke twice his size over some disputable footballing indiscretion. It was also in this game that an opponent gracefully sidestepped around Rick, our last line of defence. Rick spun around, zeroed in on the offending opponent and performed a most astonishingly ungraceful slide tackle from behind that was forever known afterwards as 'The Tackle'.

While there were only our own substitutes watching our first game against the Chefs, for our second game Jim's new girlfriend and her daughter came to cheer us on. Rick's girlfriend was also there, cheering: 'Make me proud, you big specimen!' Another friend of Jim's, Yari, also came to watch. Yari had been asked to join the team, but he'd knocked it back because he had a new baby to look after. Regardless, he got really into it while watching and had a kick-around with us at half-time.

For the rest of our games we either lost embarrassingly to teams who had really good footballers, or lost respectably (or occasionally even won or drew) to one of the other motley crews of misfits like us. Now and again we realised that maybe we were better than we thought we were – one referee actually said to Rick, 'The other team were so much better than you, but you deserved to win.'

We didn't really socialise with anyone who beat us, so that only left the Chefs to hang out with. But we got on well with them and watched their games when they didn't coincide with our own. Rick's girlfriend would shout in vain at most games: 'If you get three goals in the next five minutes you win!' But we were keen, we always turned up (once, even on a wife's birthday), always played till we couldn't play any more (two send-offs, one broken toe, one gammy back and one sprained ankle) and were always ready for a cold beer and a thorough analysis of the game afterwards. Our crowd of supporters also grew and the 'Trombettes' occasionally came to include Steve and Nick's girlfriends, my wife and my dog. But never any babies.

At the end of our regulation seven games, we finished in the bottom third of our league table by points earned – three for a win, two for a draw and one for a loss. There were three men's league tables and two women's. All the teams were then sorted by points into four groups to play the final three knock-out games (a quarter-final and possibly a semi-final and a final). The first division contained the best teams with the highest points and the fourth division contained the lesser teams with the least points. So, like every team, we still had a quarter-final to play and if we won that game we would play in a semi-final, and then if we won that we'd play in the third division grand final with a chance to win a trophy plus the surprised adulation of our partners, friends and families, and the deserved admiration of our footballing peers.

We were 2–0 down at half-time to the Matildas. We were playing on the pitch next to the canteen where all the other players met up with beers and socks down after their games had finished. At half-time, for no apparent reason, I stood up and said, 'We can do this, we have the skills.' To our astonishment, in the second half Jim scored two scorching goals, both shots from far out – the Chefs went wild on the sidelines and we felt like the Mighty Ducks doing the bobsled for Jamaica in the Winter Olympics. Near the end of full-time, Ross scored another goal, managing to fumble the ball over the line with his feet while sitting on the ground. We were 3–2 up, but only for a minute before Rick unintentionally handballed right in front of our goal. They scored. That meant the game was drawn after normal time and the rules dictated that we play on until a 'golden goal' was scored, but with each team removing one player every two minutes. It didn't make much difference to our team who we took off; we could take off everyone apart from Marcello and Jim without anyone noticing. Eventually, and predictably, they scored the golden goal and we lost. Our season ended with great pride and a little dignity.

What did we learn from that first season? Well, we learned to be humble in defeat and not to laugh at players from the other teams when they did really bad kicks. We also learned the value of filming all of our games. Usually we had seven players, so there was always someone not playing who could hold the camera. Otherwise, one of the wives or girlfriends (bless them for coming to watch at all, let alone for indulging us by helping us to film ourselves), or other fans (one of Rick's three children) would do the filming.

After our second game against the Bullfrogs, we grabbed a case of beer and returned enthusiastically to Jim's share house (next to our 'home training ground') to watch the game we had just played. We plugged the camera into Jim's TV and watched it in real-time, then in slow motion, then in real-time again. We then rewound it and watched it all over again: every brave tackle, every shot on goal that sailed way over the crossbar into the long grass behind, every save, every reaction to heckling and every goal we almost stopped from going in. The few goals that we did score were replayed so often that most of us can still remember every moment of them.

Our two halves of social football – totalling fifty minutes of 'fitness and fun' – were followed by up to six hours of drinking, carrying-on and reliving the shared experience of playing football in a team of new male friends. The team chant was invented on the front porch – 'Here they come swinging their legs, moving their feet, using their heads, they're the Rusty, they're the Rusty, they're the Rusty Trombones!' – and around the table out back we entertained each other, swapping glory stories of yesteryear. Each taking it in turn to outdo the others with a tale of bravery, heroism or stupidity. Bonding? Yes it was.

We had many messy nights at Jim's, once coming home as late as 3 a.m. Not that it stuffed up our lives the next day very often; Jim was usually surfing at 6 a.m. and Ross was on his way to work by 7 a.m. Although one night Steve left his wallet at Ross', and when Ross drove past Steve's house the next morning to drop it off, Pirate Steve answered the door on his hands and knees. Due to a back injury, he said.

After our last game of the season, we all went to the pub to watch the awards being presented to the teams that won the first, second, third and fourth division titles. The eight of us were the quiet group near the back, with the Chefs, watching in wonder and awe as the talented footballers collected their trophies. Then we piled into Rick's minibus and went back to Jim's house to watch the game we'd played that evening, the last of the season.

I guess we were all wondering when we'd see each other next, but before long Jim – as captain, coach, physio and manager – decided it would be a good idea to have an end-of-season social gathering before Christmas. We imagined this would be similar to our normal routine together, except we wouldn't play fifty minutes of football first and everyone's partner would be there. Some of us hadn't met our team mates' partners before, and they certainly hadn't all met each other. For a venue, I offered my joint and the team accepted.

Jim, Steve and Nick brought along a special DVD to watch – they had spent far too long under extraneous circumstances sitting in front of Pirate Steve's faulty computer editing together the highlights (and many lowlights) of our first season. They had added music, subtitles and commentary and had made copies for everyone, complete with covers and the following disclaimer: 'Please note some of this material is not suitable for children, WAGs and people who have no interest in watching grown men make fools of themselves in a competitive sport.'

Once again we watched ourselves perform, this time projected onto a wall – and this time in front of our wives and girlfriends. As the DVD finished, the only player who hadn't been present, Marcello, turned up. So, not unenthusiastically, we followed the same procedure as normal and watched the DVD again. Marcello loved it and asked Pirate Steve to make more copies to send to all of his friends and family back in Italy. We thought it was hilarious to watch. What at the time had felt like a powerful sprint up the sidelines spurred on by the roar of the crowd, revealed itself, in front of others, to be more like half-speed comedic running accompanied by screeches from amused onlookers. Funny sometimes how different real life feels compared to how it appears.

We all behaved a little differently that night – Rusty Trombones Lite – we certainly didn't get as toasted as we usually would on a Thursday night after playing a game together. There were dips and glasses, and it was more polite conversation than raucous camaraderie. I guess some of us were putting on something like best behaviour in front of our partners. After the second showing of the DVD, we presented Jim with a T-shirt with 'Coach' printed on it and a bunch of flowers – small, insignificant and probably inappropriate signs of our appreciation for all the work he'd put in to get us together as a team, for what was probably a one-off season of outstanding fun and accidental fitness.

By now we boys all knew each other pretty well, and on that night just before Christmas we got to know each others' partners better. Some were wives of a few years and some were girlfriends of a few months. They had been supporters of the Rusty Trombones Football Club for the season and they were deservedly part of this end-of-season, less blokey but still boozy, child-free event.

At this point, unbeknown to the rest of us, Jim and his partner, Sarah, had already started another team. He had begun his journey into fatherhood. Sarah was two months pregnant by the end of the season, but they hadn't told anyone yet and we hadn't noticed she wasn't drinking. Jim had conceived this football team and now he had conceived something much more important and life-changing. He was about to lead us into a whole new game, needing a whole new game-plan, a completely new strategy and a new set of tactics for our second season together.

Season Two

Fertile FC

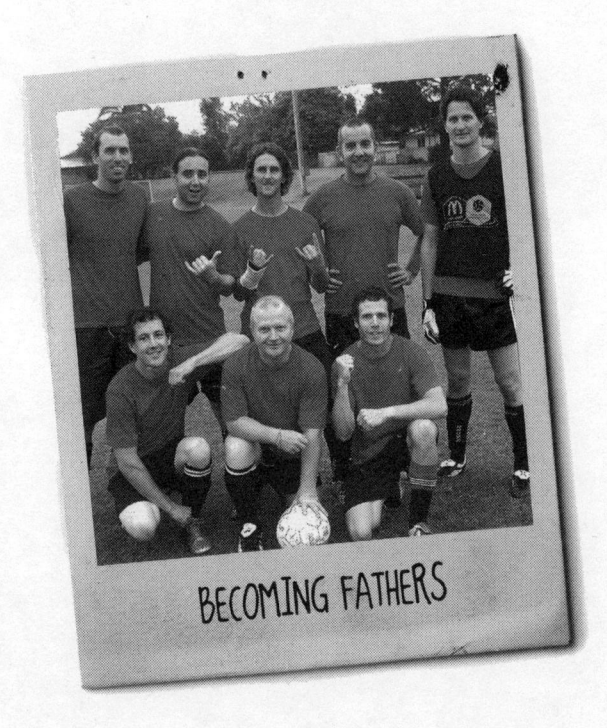

BECOMING FATHERS

FERTILE FC

JIM FIRST TOLD SOME OF US ABOUT HIS IMPENDING FATHERHOOD on New Year's Eve. He popped into Ross' house where Ross and his wife Bella, and my wife Mette and I, and other normal, non-footballing friends were all partying like it was 1999. Jim arrived with Sarah and Pirate Steve and uncharacteristically, but politely, bypassed all the drinking and smoking. He led a group of us straight out onto the back deck, where he and Sarah announced they were pregnant before heading home for a quiet night together. It was a surprise for sure; we hadn't expected this from Jim and Sarah at this stage in their new relationship, but it was clearly very good news, which made us all feel warm and fuzzy. It also made us feel alert and aware, however. Aware that the lives of those around us, and therefore our lives, were beginning to change, and alert to the fact that this could well be the last New Year's Eve celebration when we had only ourselves to try to put to bed.

It wasn't as if we shouted it from the grandstand, but Ross and Bella, and also Mette and I, had quietly let it be known that we were going to be trying for a baby after a thorough post-Christmas detox. Rick and Christina were also ready for it and 'not not trying'; and Nick was just surprised that all his new mates were so busy between games and began to worry that the consumption of beer was slipping into serious decline.

Was it strange that we were all preparing to get pregnant around the same time? We were at different ages and stages of our relationships, but all relatively settled and living where we wanted to be, with the person we wanted to be with – so maybe not. Maybe just as women's menstrual cycles align when they spend a lot of time together, so too had our reproductive urges aligned. Or maybe it was because we all felt that we now had a network of male support that would allow us to move happily onto a different stage of our lives – the final piece of the jigsaw that made the complete picture of the happy family, for each of us.

Jim's news certainly made the rest of us feel as if this really was the right time to be doing what we all seemed to be naturally considering anyway. It was like an instant, mostly unspoken, brotherhood. We pictured our kids knowing each other and growing up together, playing soccer on the same team and, who knows, maybe even one day playing together for Australia in the World Cup finals – with VIP tickets for their dads of course.

After our first six-a-side soccer season ended, we had all drifted back into our normal lives, relationships and responsibilities. Our lives were enriched by the new friendships formed, and for some of us it doubled the amount of people we knew well in the area. We didn't see each other every week anymore for football matches and story sharing, but we did begin to socialise outside football. If there were birthdays or beach parties, our new footballing friends and their partners were all invited. Through this we all indirectly met an even wider group of local people, and there were suddenly many more people to stop and chat with on a Sunday stroll through one of the local markets.

Our social circles began to mingle and overlap, and for the first time the soccer boys were invited to join the surfer boys' annual surf pilgrimage to Angourie National Park. We met up after work on a Friday and had to carry everything in – tents, food, water, beer and surfboards. It was a long hike, under a full moon, following a coastal track and deserted beaches to a little-known campsite where we'd be meeting some other surfers for a weekend in the water and on the waves. We were all fully laden, the boys with their gun boards under one arm – then came the Glaswegian and the Londoner (Ross and me), carrying a ten-foot Malibu board nose and tail through the broken scrub, up and down the rocky escarpments, over boulders and eventually along a beach to the campsite. I think we sweated more in those three hours than we did the whole football season. Yari, who'd come to watch some of our soccer games in season one, was also there, along with three or four other hardcore surfers. Sitting round the campfire at night with salt in the hair was a great time to strengthen friendships and make new mates.

As the beginning of the next six-a-side soccer season approached, Jim contacted us again to see whether we were interested in playing. I think we all knew we wanted to play, and for most of the same reasons as the year before – fitness and fun, sure, but this season wouldn't be about carrying on afterwards. Some of us had different priorities now, and besides, Jim didn't have the bachelor share house with a fridge full of beer and a vacant block next door – he was getting married and moving to a family-friendly cottage.

Twinkletoes Ezza had gone on tour around Australia working at the Big Day Out music festival, and Pirate Steve had sailed away in his home-built, thirty-foot catamaran with his two teenage sons. The team would really miss those two characters, but not really for their football skills. Someone whose football skills we would definitely miss was Marcello – he had scored all but three of our goals in the first season. He wasn't around anymore either. Rumour had it he was escorted back to Italy by customs officials, but the last we heard he was in New Zealand – probably because the girls are so beautiful in New Zealand.

That left only Jim, Rick, Ross, Nick and me, and despite the possibility of further imminent new arrivals, we decided to have another go at a season of football – but we'd have to recruit some more players. While at the beginning of our first season together the requirements to fit into the group might have been the ability to drink, stay up late and tell a good story, our situations had changed and we needed like-minded players who understood our new world order.

As season two approached, we added three new players to the team. Yari had knocked back joining the team in season one because of the birth of his first child, but now he was like a kid with candy every time someone talked about football. He'd grown up without team sport (or candy) on a commune in Nimbin but he was nothing like the dreadlocked hippy you'd expect. Yari and his partner, Nella, were busy with their young daughter, and also 'not not trying' to get pregnant with their second child. So he would find it difficult to get out once a week to play football – meaning he met all the necessary requirements.

He was extremely tall – he looked too tall for his shorts somehow – and had never played football before. But if it turned out he had absolutely no affinity for the game, at least he might look intimidating. For all his impressive stature, Yari was sweet, enthusiastic and sincere, with a hint of naivety. He was the youngest of us at twenty-nine, but he was also probably the most grown up.

'Neil, is Yari going to be there?' my partner, Mette, would ask. Ross' partner, Bella, would ask the same, and they were always happy to hear that Yari might be attending a particular social function, as there was then more chance of everyone getting home at a decent time and in one piece.

As well as Yari, there was Chad, an ex-professional snow-boarder. Yari had introduced Chad to Jim on a stealth skateboarding adventure on the newly built Brunswick Heads bridge section of the Pacific Highway the night before it opened. High on adrenaline they all went to the pub afterwards and found a common interest in football amongst the empty schooner glasses. Chad was fit, energetic like a bunny playing a drum, and had two young children. There was also Jake, another friend of Yari's and fellow collaborator of 'Frock Parties' – a popular local underground dance gathering where all the boys came in op-shop frocks. Jake was already the father of a little girl.

Jim arranged a pre-season picnic for the new players to meet the existing players and their partners, and we all met at Clarks Beach in Byron Bay. We decided to have a kick-around while the girls got to know each other better. Jim got out his ball, Chad quickly whipped off his shirt revealing his six-pack, Rick just as quickly put his shirt back on, and we played a fun, social, barefoot game.

Over the course of the off-season, to everyone's growing amazement, something strange and synchronistic happened: after Jim, first Yari, then Ross, and then Rick, and then I announced that we were pregnant (well, that our partners were pregnant – it wasn't that strange!). These weren't big announcements, but proud asides to the other boys at appropriate moments. Instead of football players whose partners happened to be pregnant, we became men whose partners were pregnant who happened to play football.

With the common denominator now being pregnant partners or new babies, as opposed to any sort of soccer skills, it seemed only fitting and appropriate that we change our team name from the Rusty Trombones FC to something else. Anything else, really. The capability of reproduction was what we proudly had in common now, and so we all agreed to rename our team 'Fertile FC'. We were acknowledging, perhaps not so covertly, the impressive and fully functioning manhood that would be hidden, but not forgotten, beneath our football shorts.

Nick was the sole bloke in the team whose partner, Sally, was not currently eating for two. He was happy for us though, and each time he heard one of us had got one past the keeper he said it felt like a team goal, and something to celebrate by running around with a shirt over his head. He didn't really speak about his own situation regarding jumping into the gene pool, and we didn't pry, but he certainly must have felt like the odd man out at some of the team talks.

For the rest of us, it was comforting and made us feel normal knowing that others were expecting babies at around the same time. It was hard to imagine being the only one of the team who became pregnant – would you change your team or your circle of friends? Would it change naturally or wouldn't it change at all? Yari and Rick had both been through the birthing and fathering adventure before, but didn't want to spoil the uniqueness of our experiences, so purposely didn't let on about the lack of sleep, lack of sex and other early paternal mysteries, and allowed the rest of us to enjoy the enthusiasm and camaraderie that was building between the dads-to-be.

We still got excited turning up at the Bangalow Sports Fields every Thursday evening. Bangalow was a quaint, one-main-street country town about ten kilometres inland from Byron Bay. It was probably best known for the local Billy Cart Derby that took place down the hill of its main street every year. It looked typically Australian; there were no large franchise or tourist shops in town, but you could still buy a Tibetan prayer mat, a Japanese kimono or an Afghan trumpet in one of the speciality stores. The sports fields had been there since the early eighties, donated by a local farmer and prepared by council earth-moving equipment from the US that arrived in Brisbane and called in at Bangalow for a test run en route to Ballina. The grounds were finished with volunteer support from the local community.

As Nick said, behind every great football team there are some very understanding women, and during the second season we saw more of the WAGs show up to join the Trombettes (still so named, the 'Fertilettes' was too weird). Christina, Bella, Sally, Nella and Mette would come and watch Rick, Ross, Nick, Yari and me play football and continue to get to know each other better. Jim's Sarah would also come to games with their new baby. Jim now drove everywhere with a huge blue inflatable exercise ball squashed against the back windows of his car. This was for Sarah to bounce gently on while nursing the baby to sleep, sometimes on the sidelines of a game.

As we now had people watching every game, we asked the partner spectators to film the football, as we had done in season one. Maybe we could get together at the end of the season to watch it? But now the filming was from Venus as opposed to Mars. While the image primarily followed the football, and the group of blokes chasing it and screaming at each other, the soundtrack was localised to the chat on the sidelines. Often the picture would pan away from the game as a pregnant partner turned up and was told how stunning she looked, or the camera would zoom in on my dog Kamu licking the opposition team substitute's leg just before he ran on. While we were exerting ourselves on the pitch, the highlights reel that year contained such footage as Chad's son singing on the sidelines; Sarah's daughter, Tallula, dancing; and only the occasional football attack into the opposition's half – and that with the unsynchronised soundtrack of female voices swapping the latest news on pregnancy, breastfeeding and evil plastics.

We probably won as many games as we lost during season two. It was the second season together for most of us and we were comfortably settling into our positions and each other's company. We also enjoyed the football more as we grew fitter and better at it. Jim broke his arm in game two after blocking a ferocious free kick, but played on for the entire game. After that he took on more of a coaching role but still came to games to ensure his emailed instructions during the week were carried out by the book. He was always there for our warm-up drill, which consisted of his dog, Asha, chasing the ball between us – we had to pass it quickly and accurately to keep the ball, and our feet, away from Asha's teeth.

We often turned up exhausted, usually had a pile of mobile phones on the sideline in case one of us got *the* call, and always went straight home after the game, either to help a heavily pregnant partner or to care for a newly arrived baby. Yari didn't miss a game, even the week Nella gave birth. Ross had his footy kit packed at home in case Bella didn't give birth on a Thursday and he could get to the game (he only missed one). Rick and I had very pregnant partners, and Jim spent more time mid-week delegating food rosters for team mates with newborns than he did organising our tactics – which already was a fair amount of time.

The meal roster was a good example of the team playing together well, off the field. After every baby was born, each player chose an evening in the first week to make the new parents a meal. We would take the meal around, have a quick visit, if convenient, to meet the new addition, then leave the family to eat their meal together. We also kept each other updated on how the parents were doing. One email from a roster organiser said: 'No need to call first, starving breastfeeding mum will eat anything (but no garlic or onions), an early drop-off would be good, 6 p.m. or so and then out coz they've had little sleep.' And then later from another deliverer of dinner: 'I went round tonight, and they WANT some visitors as they're keen to show off their new baby – stay for dinner!'

It was a way of supporting each other in the first weeks – some weeks you were cooking for others and one week they were all cooking for you. There was some pressure to prepare the most appropriate meal, not repeated and up to scratch. A list of allergies and preferences was circulated beforehand by the person organising the roster; obviously it was useful to know if someone was vegetarian or lactose intolerant. When it was Mette and my turn, I emailed the team: 'Mette: no capers. Neil: no capers, sweet potato, pumpkin, squash, olives, celery, cucumber, zucchini (or anything else that looks like cucumber), melon, fennel or hard cheeses.' This, quite rightly, received a number of obscene responses – 'Who are we cooking for here? It's the new mother who needs the attention!'

The meal roster was especially appreciated by those of us who didn't have close family nearby, and those of us who were new to the area. We were all from somewhere else, with family scattered around the country or the world. The football gave us a team, a family feeling that we shared on and off the pitch. As with football, it was all about support, being available, looking out for each other's back, and playing well together to get the best result.

After the first seven games in season two, our third-division quarter-final was against the Infarcts. Jim was playing with his arm in a plaster cast and Rick was playing with a severely bruised, almost-broken nose from an altercation with a very fast-moving, size-four leather football. We lost the game quite convincingly and once again our season was over at the first hurdle. After two more games, both without consequence as we'd lost our first qualifying quarter-final match, we went to the pub to watch the trophies being awarded to the winning teams. We presented Jim with another T-shirt (in case he'd lost the one we gave him at the end of the season before) – this time with 'One Got Past the Keeper' printed on it. Rick was designated driver that night – easy for him because Christina could have gone into labour at any moment.

Our lives were certainly changing – as they would, and certainly should, when we were experiencing something as massive as having a baby. What follows are the candid tales of conception, pregnancy and birth – the journey into fatherhood – of each of the players of our six-a-side football team around our second season. From Jim's child's birth before the season began, to Yari's, Ross', Rick's and then my baby's birth after the season finished, there were only seven months between them all. Each of us moved from footballer to father; from relative freedom to serious responsibility; from an 'I' to a 'we'; and, some would say, from a boy to a man. We were all ordinary men who, one year before, could never have imagined this would be happening to us – let alone everyone else in the team. We were connected as a football team and now that connection was about to deepen. Here are our stories.

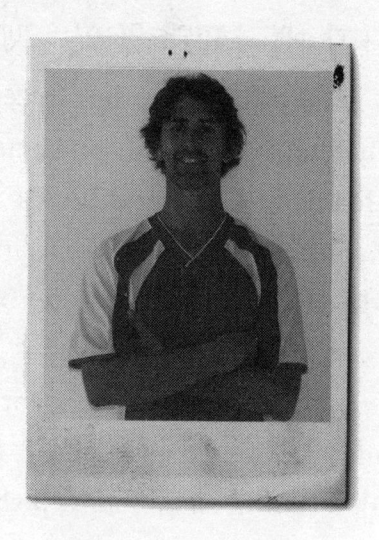

JIM'S STORY

First on the team sheet, but rarely the traditional number one of goalkeeper because he's too good in the outfield. Jim is the captain, the coach, the manager, and our best player. He can play in any position, stopping or scoring goals, or linking defence with attack. He can tackle and dribble and shout instructions (but not all at the same time). In his capacity as coach, he's a worrier, but also a visionary at understanding the flow of a game and the tactics needed to succeed. If he has a fault he's inclined to take it a bit too seriously, but his family's originally from Manchester, England, and his uncle played professionally in New Zealand, so the game is in his blood.

'COME HERE AND FEEL MY LEATHER PANTS.' THAT WAS MY LINE.

I'd been at my mate Alby's wedding reception for a few hours and was having a chat with him outside about how I'd been single for a little bit, and how I was playing the field a little bit, and why couldn't I be a little bit more like him? Why couldn't I focus my energy on meeting the right girl, someone I could share my life with – 'the One'? He'd found his 'One', and had married her that evening. It was a full moon and a star-filled night, deep in the Northern New South Wales rainforest – really lush and beautiful. Alby said, 'You'll find somebody, mate.' I smiled sadly and walked back into the hustle and noise of the party.

Previously I'd had three serious girlfriends. Serious, for me, was living together and thinking about the future together. With one – we were together for nearly seven years – we'd both wanted kids and tried to get pregnant but with no success. It bothered us enough that we went and got tested for fertility, with slightly different experiences. My experience was in a clinical, white-coat environment. It involved the scenario I'd always dreaded; getting the specimen into a little plastic cup and handing it to the lady at the front counter of the pathology lab. I quickly opened the door of my private cubicle, hurried to the counter and made 'the drop' in front of a packed waiting room. 'Thank you,' said the lady at the counter. In the same move I went for the door to make a speedy exit. 'Excuse me,' she called out after me, 'what time did you prepare the sample?' The whole room turned to look at me, and I went completely red. 'Five minutes ago,' I said sheepishly, and disappeared out the door. Definitely one of the most embarrassing moments of my life.

My partner's test consisted of going to a herbal naturopath for a consultation where they had a 'deep and meaningful' and came to the conclusion that there were too many mental blockages for her at this stage of our relationship. Funnily enough, she was spot on, and I'm glad she was. That was the catalyst for some self-analysis of our relationship and highlighted other reasons that we were not right for each other on many levels. The relationship ended a few months later.

The night of Alby's wedding, as I wound my way through the drunken revellers, I ran into Pirate Steve. He nudged me. 'Look at Sarah,' he said.

Sarah was a costume designer from Forster, four hours north of Sydney, and she was gorgeous. She struck the right chords with me, and exuded a kind of aloof confidence which I loved. She was stylish but in a natural way – unassuming not overpowering. I watched her dance in the moonlight with the other cool and confident single chicks. Luckily for me, I was a bit drunk, and I approached her with what I thought was my best smile. I used my 'leather pants' line and that was it, I was in.

The more I got to know about Sarah, the more I liked. We shared the same musical tastes and she even admitted to liking Guns N' Roses, which was a big tick in my book. And she cared. She really cared about people and this showed in her friendships and the way she treated me. She was such an earth mother, and a real mother, too, to her seven-year-old daughter, Tallula. Actually, that was one of the things that attracted me to Sarah – as well as our personal connection, being a good parent was definitely an attribute I'd been looking for in a prospective partner. I had seen her nurturing parenting style and I thought it was awesome, she treated Tallula so well in every way – she really sacrificed herself for her child.

We had never talked about having kids together – we hadn't known each other that long and had never talked about a lot of things – but after just three months, Sarah became pregnant. She'd only moved into our share house two weeks before. It was pretty full-on, but I thought, well, if it's meant to be – then bring it on. I was thirty-four.

I had a rare rush of maturity, and rather sensibly assessed whether I could be with Sarah for the rest of my life; whether we could raise kids together and whether our relationship was strong enough. Sarah had a healthy living philosophy and a healthy suspicion of some of the things that are taken for granted in western medicine. She provided Tallula with only the best organic food and natural medicines, and used the philosophies of Indigenous baby-rearing such as co-sleeping. I remember her telling me that for the first year of Tallula's life, she (or Tallula's dad) was always in the same room as her. This appealed to me. I could see Tallula was fiercely independent and I regarded this as a great character trait. One day, Sarah and I took Tallula up to stay with her granddad for a school holiday. After a brief goodbye, Tallula wandered away from us with her Pop without even a glance back to her mum – she had complete trust that she would see her mother soon and was off to have a good time.

I talked with Sarah about this on the way home and we chatted about how her parenting style, especially in the early impressionable years, had laid a good foundation for Tallula's character. She told me how she felt about 'controlled crying' and her belief that it could have a negative effect on the child's mental health in later life. She believes that babies have limited resources to ask for things, and when they cry they are not only expressing a need for nurturing from their parents, but also letting them know that there is a problem. She believes ignoring them is basically saying that their needs are not important and they can learn from that that they are not safe to express themselves. This definitely resonated with me.

I think she was unsettled by the surprise pregnancy. It was so soon after we had made the decision to commit to each other – it was a shock for both of us, for sure. Tallula was 'all grown-up now', or at least not a toddler with hourly needs, and Sarah was starting to live her life again. I also think she was scared that I would leave her and she needed constant reassurance that I wouldn't, and that everything would be okay. She didn't want to be a single mum with two children. In saying that, I could tell she was excited and happy to be pregnant, and in love. As I was.

I had already learned some valuable parenting lessons through Tallula. At first I'd struggled with the idea of coming in as a step-parent, especially to a hearing-impaired child, as Tallula is. She can be very loud and sometimes her speech is barely understandable, but she is the most inspirational and excited little child I've ever met. She takes the world on headfirst and doesn't look back. She is a real character. She uses sign language to communicate, so I booked into TAFE and did a one-year signing course. I think it really helped our relationship to grow – it gave me a much better understanding of Tallula and the skills to communicate with her properly.

I'd hardly had any experience with kids before – only cousins in New Zealand, and briefly mentoring two boys through Uncle, a program for boys without active fathers (but that only involved taking them skating or surfing). I found it all a bit daunting – but Tallula taught me a lot. The biggest thing you find out about being a parent is that you have to learn to be unselfish: 'Okay, you selfish bastard, it's not about you now, she's a child and you have to look after her no matter what.' Once I told myself this it became so obvious. It wasn't easy to keep that line of thought though – the selfish thoughts were constantly knocking at the door, asking to come back in and be trusted again, like an unfaithful ex-partner. Sure, I'd rather have spent my money on a surfing trip to Indonesia than on horse-riding outings, but once you've committed yourself to someone else, you know it's the way to be and it becomes easier to leave the selfish thoughts outside in the rain. It just wasn't all about me anymore.

It was around this time that the idea of conceiving a football team was bounced around. My ex-flatmate Marcello had moved out to be with his partner in Byron Bay, but before he went, we had discussed forming a soccer team for the Summer Sixes six-a-side competition, which he had played in during the previous off-season. Being the Italian stallion he was, he had issues with being subbed off – he wanted to play the entire game. I suggested that we start our own team and make our own rules – he could play the whole game all the time, and he enthusiastically agreed. Marcello had come from Italy and used his time while travelling around Australia to hone his football-juggling skills. He had toured the country busking with a drummer: the drummer drummed while he juggled the soccer ball and did a number of fancy tricks, which eventually earned him the nickname 'Fancyfoot'.

So the idea was born. The next step was enlisting some more players. My friend Ezza had just broken up with his partner of twelve years and was living in the area at my suggestion. He was working occasionally with another friend of mine, Steve, who had a building business. The three of us had formed a trio of mateship. We were all trying to get fit – doing laps at the pool and surfing – so when I suggested the idea of playing soccer they had no hesitation, even though they had never played the game before. So I had four players and the beginning of a team, of sorts. I just needed another four or five players. I started asking some of my other friends, some I had known for a while and some I hadn't. I asked Neil, Ross and Rick, and to my surprise they were all keen to play. A team was born.

I was feeling good, my life was coming together and we were going to have a baby. I had a rush of happy, self-centred testosterone – 'My swimmers do work!' – which felt pretty good after trying for so long to get pregnant in my last relationship and thinking maybe I could never have a child, despite what the fertility test had told me. I was stoked, but then my guts went 'holy shit!', as I started to think about the consequences of responsibility: looking after a kid; not being single, free and easy anymore; not going for a surf whenever I wanted – this was going to be pretty full on. I was confident I could do it, but there were a lot of questions that I began to ask myself over the following weeks. Then, after eight weeks, Sarah lost the baby.

I was at work. Sarah phoned to say that something was wrong and she was going to see the doctor. When I got home, she'd had a scan and even though she'd started bleeding, the doctor said it was still okay and to take it easy. Through the night the situation worsened and by the next morning we went for another scan to confirm what we already knew.

We had told a few close friends and family we were pregnant when we found out at eight weeks, even though it's not really the done thing. I had heard about the twelve-week rule – people don't generally tell others that they are pregnant in the first twelve weeks, because that's when most miscarriages happen – but we felt we needed the support.

Shamefully, I was a little bit pissed off. We'd made this major decision to have a baby, even though we hadn't known each other for very long, and I was ready now. Sarah was devastated: sick, angry, emotional and slightly depressed. I was probably less supportive than I could have been, as I was going through a myriad of emotions as well. We had a big argument and I think it was the culmination of all the stress around the miscarriage that made us go at each other so hard. It was probably my fault – I just didn't understand why everything had happened the way it had.

About a month after that we decided to call it quits. Sarah went to a Vipassana retreat and took a vow of silence for ten days. I went to stay with a close friend, Chewie, and talked all day and all night. I told Chewie I thought I was losing the one person I could be with; that I was terrified of losing her, but that there were some things that were confronting about our relationship – such as being a step-parent – that were skewing my normal thought processes. I told him I thought Sarah and I connected so well and shared so many things in common. I told him openly and honestly what was on my mind and eventually he said, 'She's "the One", mate.' After talking to my mum, who agreed with Chewie, I agreed with both of them.

Within the space of a month, Sarah and I were back together. She had returned from the retreat vibrant and with a new air of self-confidence and sense of self. She came over to my place not long after she got back and told me that she always knew that we were meant to be, but that I'd needed to figure that out in my own time. It had taken me about two hours. I was smitten all over again. And it didn't take long before we were pregnant again.

When Sarah told me the news I became angry, which I regretted later. We'd decided to wait before trying again; to take the opportunity to be together as a couple and cement our relationship; to get some savings together. The doctor had told us that after a miscarriage it takes at least three months for the female body to even start contemplating reproduction again. We thought we were safe. We were wrong.

I guess that was why I was a little bit angry. I am the sort of person that needs order in my life – I'm a Taurean, for God's sake, we don't like change, and here I was with my world being thrown into chaos. I've always believed that things come along when they're supposed to, that everything happens for a reason, but let's just say I wasn't jumping for joy. It was more like, 'Why couldn't this have happened six months down the track?' Sarah, of course, was a bit upset with this attitude, which caused some friction, but I came around soon after by having a stern word with myself.

At this time we were about four games into the first season as the Rusty Trombones FC and having plenty of laughs on and off the field. I was really enjoying playing, although I was apprehensive about my weak ankles, which is why I had originally stopped playing football a few years prior. I had sprained my ankles so many times while playing soccer and skateboarding that I had lost count. The last straw was while playing in Sydney for Maroubra United; I was running around the training pitch for a warm up, stood on a pine cone, and heard a massive snap in my ankle. I was laid up for two weeks to recover – and I was only in my late twenties.

I had played a lot of soccer in my younger years before I found girls, rock and skateboarding at around eighteen. My uncle had played for the All Whites and my family was soccer mad, so all family gatherings centred on a game of soccer in the backyard. I also played competitively after university, but the teams I played for took it very seriously. I guess that's what I liked about forming the Rusty Trombones – the opportunity to have a team made up of members who connected on a personal level and liked to have some laughs. I definitely enjoyed getting to know the lads and having that regular outlet for socialising. I think it really allowed everyone to let their hair down.

The guys would all come over to my house after the games and we'd drink beers. I knew that this was my last hoorah and that by the end of the season I would need to be taking serious care of Sarah, and myself. I also wished I could have shared what I was going through with the lads from the team, but I didn't want to create false expectations again. I sure as hell didn't want to show too much happiness in case it went bad.

I couldn't let myself believe it was actually going to happen, I couldn't put energy into it, not again, not until it was sure. It didn't seem long ago – it wasn't long ago – that I was telling family and getting excited and I couldn't stand having that all fall in a heap again. So I got smart about it. I learned a lot about positive wellbeing and good health from a naturopath GP. I realised Sarah was going to put her body under a lot of stress and she had to become as healthy as she could. I needed to take care of her. She followed an eating plan, had blood tests, ate iron-rich foods, did whatever we learned was necessary so that we would have the best chance possible.

There are two things I remember above all else about the first trimester (the first three months of pregnancy). First, Sarah was so sick that she couldn't get out of bed in the morning. If I didn't get some food into her before her feet hit the floor at 5.30 a.m. – and not just any food, it had to be avocado spread thickly on sweet-and-sour rye bread with a little Promite – then it was nausea and vomiting for the rest of the day.

Secondly, I remember the first scan at twelve weeks. This is the first-trimester scan; a 'nuchal translucency' scan usually done between about eleven and thirteen weeks. The main reason for this scan is to work out if the foetus is likely to have a chromosomal abnormality, such as Down syndrome, but it can also reveal other conditions. Once we were given the all clear, we could start to tell family and friends that we were past the most common time to miscarry. We told our families on Christmas Eve, which was the best present we could have given them.

The first football season ended in the second week of December. We celebrated with an end-of-season party at Neil's house and the lads gave me some flowers. We watched the season-highlights video and I was filled with pride with what we'd created on the field. It had been a great season with lots of good times, fun and frivolity. I knew I wouldn't see some of these guys again on the football field so I had cherished the time spent playing, knowing that Sarah was resting comfortably at home. I think the end of the first season became the start of a whole new way of life for me as my priorities changed from nurturing a football team of blokes to nurturing Sarah and my new family.

As soon as Sarah was 'properly' pregnant, I started to forget about football and began worrying about having a healthy baby. Was my baby going to be all there? If not, could I handle caring for a child with disabilities? Tallula was profoundly deaf and I knew how much extra work it was to take care of her. My father's cousin had severe cerebral palsy and I grew up seeing the workload and stresses that put on Dad's aunt. The rewards are great, don't get me wrong, but it is undoubtedly harder work and more stressful. I wasn't sure I was capable of handling that situation and it worried me. What quality of life would a child like that have? Would we have? Would I have?

It was at about this time, not long after the end of our first football season, that I joined the library at a local baby shop and started to read to find out more about what was going on in Sarah's body. I also read books and material on the internet about how a new baby would affect eight-year-old Tallula. We gave her a book on the subject, *What's Inside Your Tummy, Mummy?*, and I think it helped give her some ownership of the pregnancy and started her thinking about her role as a big sister.

Another book I found useful was *The Magical Child*. One night at dinner, Sarah said, 'You have to read this book, this is how I parent.' She went on to say she was happy to discuss and consider other styles of parenting if I brought something to the table with research, but not until I'd read this book to see where she was coming from. I hadn't really thought about styles of parenting I guess, and I thought it was pretty cool to be considering it. I have to say, I thought the book was absolute nonsense at first, but after about the first fifty pages, it started to make sense to me. It was a bit out there in its alternative views – saying that the bright lights and western lifestyle in general are too much for a newborn baby. After reading it, I asked Sarah a lot of questions, we discussed it, and I came around to her way of thinking. Like her parenting style, she was going to do the birth her way, she had certain ideas and I was going to support that – after all, she was the one who had to go through it.

The other thing we discussed early on, and another book I read on Sarah's advice, was about vaccination – *Vaccination Roulette*. I knew that Sarah didn't want to vaccinate our baby, and after I read that book I understood why. Although it felt as if there was not enough evidence either way, and that the stats were always skewed in favour of whatever bias I was reading, the stories of real people experiencing severe trauma with their child within hours of vaccinating helped me make my decision. It's not that I'm against vaccinating in principle but Sarah felt really strongly about it and I would have had to bring a hell of a lot of research and evidence to the table to win her over on this one. There is a lot of information out there on this topic, and I think it's important for everyone to come to their own conclusion as to what is best for their family.

Everyone told me – friends and family told me, mothers of experience and reputation told me, naturopaths and midwife friends told me, even Sarah told me – that the second trimester was going to be easier. After fourteen weeks the sickness stops. Stops. It's all over. You'll be on easy street.

So I circled it on my calendar, set an alarm on my phone and awaited the happy day. At fifteen weeks – I thought maybe it's a week late. Sixteen weeks. Eighteen weeks. It just didn't friggin' stop. While Sarah's first pregnancy had been fine, for this pregnancy she was sick the entire time. The *entire* time. Up to and including the childbirth. I've heard people say – and I don't know if it's true, but I've heard from friends who've experienced the same thing – that after a miscarriage, the body makes up for it by overcompensating with the hormones to ensure a healthy pregnancy the next time around. As I said, I don't know if it's true, but it felt as though Sarah's body wasn't going to let this one go easily. The baby was getting all the good stuff, we reasoned, and that's why Sarah was so sick.

At the eighteen-week scan we found out it was a girl. Initially, I was a little disappointed. I guess deep down I wanted a boy to play football with – but that was the selfish (and sexist) thoughts shouting in my head again. Also, the antiquated idea about male heirs to carry on propagating the genes was somehow stuck in my evolutionary-driven mindset. And I used to be a boy (some say I still am), I knew what that was like, but a girl? I already pictured myself as the father with the shotgun threatening the boyfriend on the front porch – 'What are your intentions towards my daughter, boy?' I was going to be that guy.

The eighteen-week scan was on an old machine at a nearby rural hospital, and it broke down halfway through, giving us just enough time to determine the gender but nothing else. We were advised to have another scan at twenty weeks because the sonographer had seen what he thought was a 'two-vessel cord'. A two-vessel cord! What? How many are there supposed to be?

I got home and googled 'two-vessel cord' and started freaking out immediately. Basically, a quarter of all babies born with a two-vessel cord (instead of the normal three vessels) have deformities or are stillborn. If I wasn't before, I was now in a state of complete fear for the rest of the pregnancy. The only thing that calmed me down slightly was the excellent sonographer at our twenty-week scan, who said he'd seen heaps of these before and that the baby comes out all right.

'Healthy baby', 'healthy baby', were the words that kept nagging away in the back of my head, and the more internet research I did, the worse my fears became. If only I hadn't known all this stuff, I'm sure I wouldn't have been as worried. A couple we knew had decided to take this a step further and have no scans throughout the pregnancy – they felt that whatever happens, happens. I'm not that person – I need to know. But I wish I didn't.

I did not really enjoy the pregnancy as much as I could have because of that. I couldn't relax. We couldn't relax. Sarah was to have another scan (her fourth) at thirty-two weeks; this was done especially to check if there were any further complications with the baby due to the two-vessel cord. It was not until this scan that we knew everything was good and that the baby was healthy.

Except, at the thirty-two-week scan, we found out the baby was now breech. What is that? I found out it means that the baby is in a bum-down, head-up position and that if it didn't turn round before birth we might need a caesarean birth rather than a natural one. Now, like I said before, Sarah has a healthy suspicion of the western medical approach. She had a good natural birth with Tallula and didn't want to undergo a hospital procedure for the birth of her second child – I didn't much like the sound of the big needle thing either – so we looked at our options. Here we go again, I thought, if it's not one thing it's another. To naturally turn the baby, Sarah tried acupuncture and swimming. And, with six weeks to go, the baby turned around – hallelujah! We're nearly there. Please, aren't we?

While Sarah was pregnant, I went away once on a surfing-safari weekend with some old surfing buddies and some new soccer mates. This was a good time outside my normal routine to reflect on what was happening at home. It was during this trip, around the campfire with all the other lads, that Yari told me he was having another baby. It was a great weekend and set me up to be in the right mind space for the final few weeks of the pregnancy. I returned refreshed and ready.

Both Sarah and I had attended 'Preparation for Childbirth and Early Parenthood' pre-natal classes supplied free by our local community-health department (two hours, one night a week, for seven consecutive weeks). These were very helpful for me. On the first evening, as an ice-breaker we went around the room introducing ourselves. About fifteen to twenty minutes in, I realised everyone in the room was in the same boat – that they were all stressing as much as me. Sarah was pretty relaxed because she'd already had a child, but before that evening (because of the two-vessel cord and breech alarms) I thought I was the most stressed-out person in the world. Turned out some of the women in this group were worse than me. And further, most of the blokes were even worse than them. They were all fidgety and uncomfortable and I suddenly understood that it was normal and okay to be worried and fearful even. There was only one bloke who was really relaxed; he slept through most of the classes he came to, but I found out that he already had five kids.

There were about twelve couples, and on the first night all but one father-to-be was there. But by the fourth week there were only three of us, and by the sixth week, only one of me. I was the only partner who attended all seven classes. It was great for me, it settled my nerves. I found out heaps about things I hadn't even thought of before: nappies, breastfeeding – none of the other men turned up for that one – I thought it was really good. Previously, I had thought you got the baby, and – bang – straight onto the boob. But, my friends, let me tell you, it's not that way at all. There are positions, angles, techniques – fingers are involved – and yet it's made out to be the most natural thing in the world.

The one thing I couldn't stomach was the video of a woman actually giving birth. I pretended I had to go to the toilet. Sarah didn't want to see it either, she left to go to the toilet too, but it was occupied.

It was also at these classes that I learned what is meant by a 'vaginal show' – and disappointingly it wasn't what I thought at all. It's when mucus presents itself from the vagina to show that the process of labour is not far off. I learned this when, at one class, we played a game in which the midwife gave us all a card describing a birth topic, such as 'waters break'. We had to decide whether the condition on our card warranted a trip to the hospital or whether you should stay at home: for example, when the waters break you stay at home. Well, it turned out, in a full class, I got the last card – vaginal show! I was slightly embarrassed and the whole class began to chuckle. I guessed correctly that this was a stay-at-home condition (wouldn't any man stay home for a vaginal show, I thought). After that, it became a running joke between Sarah and me: as the due date drew closer, every conversation or SMS was prefaced by 'is it show time'?

We were getting close now, and we had prepared a pretty comprehensive birth plan – a list of our preferences for the birth – which we were encouraged to put together at the childbirth classes. We didn't want vaccinations or interventions (unless the doctor or midwife talked to me first). We'd chosen to have our baby at the local natural-birthing centre and had some aromatic oils and comfort rugs to take into our private room. Sarah only wanted soft light, no harsh glare. A copy of our birth plan was given to the midwives, but I don't think they read it all, just the sections that were important to them – no interventions and no vaccinations. We also gave a copy to our support person, Sally, a friend of Sarah's who would be with us throughout the time we were at the birthing centre. We chose Sally because she is a naturopath and is such a nurturing person and friend.

As the day approached, I felt ready. Secretly, I wanted to get it over with. I was a bit apprehensive of course, but wanted it over so much as I'd been stressed out for so long now. It was about 8 a.m. and I'd gone into work for an hour to fill out a rental application for a new house when I got the call from Sarah – 'My waters have broken!' Her waters breaking was the sign that we were starting labour and the birthing process. The women I worked with started freaking out: 'What? She's called and her waters have broken? Get outta here!' But I was cool about it, I knew from the classes that there was no big hurry. I completed the rental application, dropped it into the real estate agent's on the way home and called my mum to tell her the news. She lived in Brisbane but said she would drop everything and get down here as soon as possible to help out (after all, it was her first grandchild and she was very excited).

Once I arrived home, by this stage late morning, we got everything ready and packed the car, and then walked together, my mum included, the short distance into the township to buy supplies. We'd been told that walking is helpful for women in labour and can speed up the process. We walked into town again in the early evening, waiting for the contractions to shorten to around seven to ten minutes apart. We knew from pre-natal classes, and from Sarah's previous birthing experience, that we just had to wait before going to the birthing centre – there was no point getting there too early. We rang them anyway to tell them we were nearly ready. We also rang Sally to tell her we were going home to bed to wait.

By about 9.30 p.m., Sarah was fully contracting and Sally and her boyfriend Nick came over to support us. Nick was the left-back for the Rusty Trombones. He had brought a copy of the charming book *All Creatures Great and Small* by James Herriot and thought it might be relaxing for us to have him read it aloud. Grateful as we were, the heart-warming and often hilarious adventures of a country veterinarian in post-war England – which included testing cows for tuberculosis and stitching up a dog's genitalia – weren't doing it for Sarah or me at this particular moment of our lives. I remember looking across the room at Nick while he was reading, and thinking, What are you *doing*?

Sarah looked at me, and I said to her, 'I think we should go to the birthing centre, what do you reckon?' So we went to a quieter place where no one was reading about Dr James Herriot struggling on the cobblestone floor of a dilapidated barn in the middle of a wintry night, with his arm up a cow.

I thought I was doing a pretty good job so far – better than Dr Herriot, anyway – I was massaging, hugging and encouraging. Before we left home we'd rung the birthing centre and asked them to fill one of the birthing baths that were available. But on this particular evening – for the first time in the proud history of the birthing centre – they had no hot water. So when we arrived, Sally and I started running buckets of hot water from the kitchen to the bath like the sorcerer's apprentices – here we go again, again! By now it was getting late into the night and Sarah was reeling in pain – not screaming though, she said her Vipassana silence retreat helped her to cope with the pain.

At about 6.30, in the early morning light, I was in the bath with Sarah and she was not coping well. She had been pushing and pushing and vomiting all night long and was worn out. I could feel my 'there must be something wrong' notion welling inside and I was beginning to second-guess everything, when at that moment the midwives changed shift and the new midwife changed tack with us.

Sarah said in her exhaustion, 'I don't think I can do it, something doesn't feel right.' Knowing Sarah, I understood that this meant she really couldn't do it. I gestured to the doctor and firmly asked, 'Could there be something wrong?' I'm glad I did. After speaking with the doctor, the midwife asked Sarah if she could intervene to check that she was fully dilated. She discovered the baby's head was caught on the lip of the cervix. Sarah had to push hard one last time while the midwife held the cervix back, and Bijou Emily was born ten minutes later in the warm bath.

I immediately freaked out. 'Look at the size of her feet. Look at her hands – they're huge!' I had read that club feet and oversized hands (and cleft palates) were common with two-vessel cords. I was frantically searching the baby's limbs and couldn't enjoy the moment at all. I looked at the doctor. 'She's fine, mate.' I still didn't believe him.

Then they suctioned the baby, putting tubes inside her mouth – they didn't ask us about that, but she wasn't breathing very well when she came out, so I guess that's something they have to do. The umbilical cord was pulsing, and wasn't cut for about forty minutes – it may have only had two vessels but those two sure worked well. Bijou hadn't cried yet, and when she was placed on Sarah's stomach, the little thing fell asleep straight away. When she eventually woke up, she immediately started to look for the nipple, which she soon found. That was such a beautiful moment. I remember when I saw my younger brother not long after he'd been born and he looked squished, spotty and red in the face – but Bijou came out perfect.

It was a total relief. From serious stress to absolute joy in seconds. Really cool. The rest of the day was pure euphoria. I remember thinking that it was the best thing that'd ever happened to me. Better than the great goals I'd scored, better than the great waves I'd caught – seriously, it was better than them all.

I panicked a little the first time I held Bijou – that was probably after about an hour. Then at about 2 p.m. a screaming woman was brought into the birthing centre. She was swearing and carrying on, and she was in the room next to us. Our new-found bliss didn't need this particular soundscape, and Sarah wanted to get out. So we left the birthing centre about six hours after the birth and went home.

Both my mother and Sarah's were at our house waiting, and having downed two expensive bottles of champagne they were well tipsy. As soon as we arrived home, Sarah's father, Sally and Nick also joined the celebrations with a bottle or two. It's weird, because you can't do anything except stare at the baby. Everyone in the room just quietly stood around looking at the baby. After nine or ten months of pure agony, you're all just there, all day, looking at this thing that doesn't do anything. Surreal.

I don't remember the first night – day and night blurred together, but I know we all slept in the same bed. The first week we were in bed most of the time, like John and Yoko. I don't think Bijou ever slept in the middle, because I was scared of sleeping next to her and rolling on her. Also, she woke every hour anyway, so we didn't really get any good sleep. Our families were visiting and staying locally, so for those first few days we didn't have any time on our own. It was frenetic, but they were all helpful – cooking and cleaning and, of course, just looking at the baby. It was quite crowded, but that was a good thing; I liked having a mob around celebrating the birth. I liked it for Bijou, for her to be surrounded by all these people who are her family. I wanted it to be social and for her to be a part of it, as well as the reason for it.

Some of the football team popped round with dinner over the first few nights, which was greatly appreciated. Yari had first raised the idea of a food roster for me and offered to organise the whole thing for us. Fittingly, it was his partner Nella's moussaka that resonates on my taste buds to this day. Neil and Mette also dropped off some food and stayed to stare at Bijou for a while, and I became somewhat emotional at the fact that all my friends were supporting us in this way – it was wonderful.

Since then, actually having a baby has been hard work. It's emotionally draining, a battle in every sense, and I certainly wasn't prepared for it. Everyone tells you it's harder than you think but, as Neil wryly said later of his first few weeks, 'Nobody told me it wouldn't be fun!' It's the hardest job I've ever had. It consumes every bit of my being. I'm always thinking about it. The sleep deprivation is the worst thing

– it's aged and wearied me. The only way we could get our daughter to sleep was on a huge bouncy ball – one of those fitness balls that can be used as an ergonomic chair. Sarah was so tired one evening, she sat on the ball while trying to get the baby to sleep and it worked. So then we took the ball everywhere with us, like an inflatable pet. This huge, blue, bouncy ball was constantly in the back of the car, with us all day, and then taken out with Bijou's baby bag when we arrived home again. It was the only way she would go to sleep. She hated the car seat. 'All babies like car seats', we heard. Well, this baby didn't. I wished she bloody well did, but she didn't.

It's not only looking after a baby, but it's looking after a mother too – you become a support person, fetching and carrying on demand. And you're new to it. Going back to work was fantastic, it was my respite from the constant caring, although I still felt bad for Sarah because she was working so hard all the time with Bijou. Of course, she had her hormones running hot and had a different connection with the baby. It was a challenge to the relationship as well. You have to change your expectation of what your relationship is – you might get an hour to yourselves and then you go, 'Wow!' That doesn't mean you're going out dancing or getting pissed; you might do a crossword in that hour and it's like heaven on earth.

The flip side is that it's the best thing you've ever done in your whole life. You suddenly have purpose and responsibility. This little thing looks at you and loves you unconditionally whatever you do. Does it get better as it goes on? I don't know that it gets better, but it gets easier. Certain moments, I think, This is the best time – right now, and then a few days later: Right now, *this* is the best time. It's a constantly changing thing. My mother once said to me that my brother and I were the best things she ever did. 'What are you talking about?' I said. 'Surely going to Greece, or having five weeks holiday from work were the best things, not me and my brother.' But now I totally understand. That's the other good thing about it – you connect with every other person in the world who has ever had a baby. You know the stuff they've been through, the joy they've had and the effort they've put into it. I'd be sorry now if I had never done it.

After a few weeks we gradually settled into our new routine and accepted 'time poor' as the new time. Gradually, I managed to think a little about football, mostly while at work. A new season of Summer Sixes would start in a few months and it was time to get the team back together – if the others were up for it. I knew we'd need a few more players as some of the guys had moved away from the area. Would it be the same now? Would I be the same with the other guys? Would they be the same with me? Had I changed?

Tallula loved having a little sister. She adored Bijou, without a hint of jealousy. The only two real difficulties for her were the sudden need to share her mother's attention, which she'd had a complete monopoly on for seven years, and the fact that Bijou was extremely sensitive to loud noises. For a deaf child, this was disastrous. On a daily basis, poor Tallulu was being reminded to lower the volume of her voice, which was very frustrating for her.

The one piece of advice I'd offer to anyone about to embark on the journey into fatherhood is, 'Look after your woman.' Sacrifice yourself because she's giving you something amazing. I appreciate and cherish the time we spent together before the baby came along, and I realise now that it might be five or ten years before we have that again. What you do beforehand with your partner to build a good relationship will make you strong through the hard work of having and nursing a baby.

Also, don't push your ideas and opinions onto others, 'You should/shouldn't read/do this' are just not cool things to say. We found initially, and understandably, that both sets of our parents had ideas about what was right and what was wrong. We were given a lot of advice and opinions, particularly on vaccination and sleeping practices. They sent information supporting the way they thought about things, but I sent back information that supported the way we thought about things. I guess they cancelled each other out because I didn't often hear back again. Obviously, our parents had been through it before and did a pretty good job – which is why I'm here to tell this story – but if we said something contrary to what they thought, then it seemed like we were judging their parenting style, which of course we weren't.

Would I do it again? Right now, I'd have to say no, as I'm completely worn out, and luckily Sarah doesn't want to either. I don't think I could cope with all the worry and stress again. I can understand why people have two babies almost back-to-back and get it over with.

A bloke Ross knew told him it was best to have two kids close together if you were going to have a second. He said it's like having two guys wanting to fight with you in the pub and one guy takes you outside and gives you a kicking. He reckons you might as well go back into the pub and get the other guy to come out and bash you too, rather than coming back another night and getting the same. I don't know if I entirely agree with how he sees the world, but I know what he means.

You do forget about all the bad things over time, people with heaps of kids say you forget, that's why you do it again.

Every day of my life has changed now. Just waking up in the morning and seeing Bijou smile or come in for a hug is melt-in-the-mouth stuff. And I'm finding all sorts of new challenges as I become more engaged with her. I'm now dealing with my own insecurities and the failings I have as a person and worrying whether my daughter will appreciate and accept me with these faults. Will this little person like me for who I am with all my weaknesses? Some people don't get on with their parents, where does that go wrong? How does it change? They loved each other once when they were little. I hope we can stay connected as she grows older.

After the baby was born, I felt like a grown-up – like a real adult. Yes, I feel like I've finally grown up. I had been proud of getting a group of blokes together to become a football team, and become friends, but that was nothing compared with how proud I felt becoming a father.

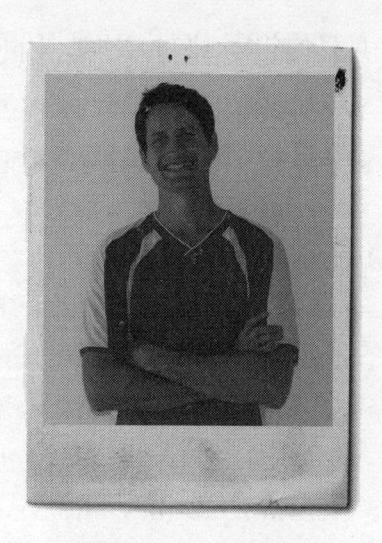

YARI'S STORY

A tall defender, or striker, who can head the ball well and has a good right foot. Not encouraged to play team sports as a child, Yari is new to the game as an adult but has become a natural player through watching lots of football and playing as much as he can. A cautious thinker and planner - as a player and as a person - he has brought strength, aggression and self-belief to his game as he's become more comfortable on the pitch and has proved himself a valuable addition to Fertile FC.

GROWING UP ON A COMMUNE NEAR NIMBIN REALLY INFLUENCED my ideas about parenting. Running wild in the hills with dozens of kids I called my half-brothers and sisters, we had the freedom to do whatever we wanted, in a really safe environment. My parents had emigrated from Germany in 1981 when I was just three to live the hippy dream on thirty acres in Nimbin, a small dairy town in Northern New South Wales, known as Australia's hippy capital after the 1973 Aquarius Festival. We were joined by up to sixteen other German families and visitors in our ex-army tents, makeshift kitchen shack and new-found warm Australian outdoor lifestyle. We ground our own flour, baked bread communally and made cheese from our goat's milk. We had no hot water (unless we fired up the same oven that cooked our bread and heated a forty-four gallon drum of water) and bathed in two old cast-iron bathtubs under the stars. No electricity, no washing machine and definitely no TV.

We would roam in ever-changing packs of kids to the local water holes, swimming nude and eating wild passionfruit, mangoes and persimmons. We had a healthy idea of body image and real examples of what girls looked like as we all hit puberty together.

Often I would stay with friends at Tuntable Falls, a huge community with two hundred members. We would get dropped off from the bus and the girls would whistle for their horses, jump on bareback and ride home, with a friend or two on the back. The boys would have to walk, or if they were lucky they'd have a motorbike and race the girls home.

As kids on a commune, we could drop into nearly any house on the 1200-odd acres and any other parent would feed, look out for, and discipline us (verbally only, no one was allowed to hit the kids). It was a very shared-parenting style, and I can see now how much easier it was for our parents living in a community and sharing so many of the small tasks that become repetitive and mind-numbing in a 'normal' modern family.

As an adult, I always thought that I'd have children of my own. But when and who with? I was living near Byron Bay in a Suffolk Park surfer share house with a great bunch of single guys and working as a web designer. I was in my mid-twenties and was starting to get over the dating thing, and then bam! I met the most happy, gorgeous and adventurous woman while sitting around a backyard bonfire at a party. It was love at first sight.

Narelle or, as she prefers, Nella, came from Grafton. She was a country girl who outgrew the small country-town life and, apart from some years studying in Sydney and Wollongong, spent most of her youth travelling the world searching for the next adventure. When I looked across the backyard bonfire that night, I saw the biggest, happiest smile on this cute blond girl and I thought, If I don't go over there now, I'll miss the best chance I may ever have.

Normally I would have been really shy in that situation, but luckily I'd made a 'love pact' with my two single flatmates to ask at least one girl out on a date every week. Yes, every week. That's at least fifty-two girls a year! It seemed impossible at first, but we rose to the challenge and were approaching the opposite sex at record pace. At one stage we even upped our challenge to twice a week. That's over a hundred girls a year, if we lasted! It wasn't about going on fantastic dates or getting loads of sex, it was more a chance for us to soothe our jangled nerves and get used to approaching girls and talking to them. It had been only maybe a month, but I'd become quite good at being myself, without the nerves, when talking to pretty girls I didn't know.

And so I gathered my courage and went and spoke to Nella. We immediately got talking about a surf trip to Mexico that she was planning. I remember being so impressed with her sense of adventure. She surfed, and had recently quit her job as a dietician at Lismore Base Hospital to start her own business. Nothing seemed too big or unachievable for her, and she had a great sense of timing. Before juice bars popped up in every shopping mall, there was 'The Juice Bus', her funky, bright yellow, converted kombi-van selling fresh juices and smoothies at the beaches of Byron Bay.

We managed to sneak in a short coffee date before I left for a two-week holiday, and as soon as I arrived back I invited her out for dinner. I couldn't wait to get to know this fun-loving, gutsy country girl. Nella was thirty-two, and I was a tender twenty-six.

We did talk about having kids about three months into the relationship. We both wanted them at some point in the future but not for at least two or three years, and we planned to have a lot of fun together before then. We wanted to enjoy our lifestyle in Bryon, go travelling – surfing in Mexico, working in the UK, visiting my family in Germany, Spain, Italy, the world! One day we took a picnic up to the Cape Byron lighthouse and under a full moon we sketched out rough plans for a trip to Europe. We planned and saved and dreamed of our future.

During this time the sex was great; it was very passionate and we spent months in each other's arms and bedrooms. I think it became a bit of a running joke for our flatmates. I'd come over and the door to Nella's room would shut and we'd only come out to eat and swim in the pool, then straight back into the bedroom.

After only a few short months of this bliss, we had a pregnancy scare. It was a huge shock for both of us – it just wasn't the right time, we both agreed. We were having so much fun. All of our travel plans would have to be cancelled. Our next few fun and carefree years together would have to be cancelled too. I knew how hard it was raising children, having spent a lot of time with my sister who was just twenty when she had her daughter, Tameeka. All the things you slowly give up: friendship, time for your own life and plans. It just wasn't the time for us. We wanted to have kids, but not now.

It turned out to be a false alarm, but from then on sex was very different. We were compulsive with condoms, paranoid about the tracking of her cycle and obsessive about withdrawal. The pill didn't agree with Nella, she questioned what it did to her body, using synthetic hormones to alter the natural reproductive rhythm. We wouldn't have sex for three or four days before we thought Nella would be fertile, and we wouldn't have sex for three or four days after, either. It felt like this left us with only a few days a month when we could have sex.

Before our big 'beer-and-cheese-fuelled European trip', Nella moved in with me for six weeks to save money. We gave away the little furniture we had and started out on our overseas trip. We had been together for one year at this point. Nella desperately wanted to live in Spain, so she went ahead to find an apartment while I followed three days later after visiting my cousins in Munich.

The day I arrived in Seville was really hot, it was the middle of summer when most people have the sense to stay away and most of the locals shut down their businesses. Spain felt new and different; such a passionate culture of food and animated language. I was happy to think that Seville was where I was going to live for a while even as I wandered lost down the narrow streets on that first day. By sheer luck I ran straight into Nella and we had a big hug, then she began to cry. She was sobbing all the way back to our new apartment, and when we got there she broke down and told me she was pregnant. This was a big surprise. We worked out we must have conceived while we were trying so hard not to with all our precautions. I was shocked, but mostly genuinely happy. We spent a whole month in Spain un-planning all the things we'd planned and getting used to the idea that we would be parents.

The first three months of this first pregnancy were tough. Nella was always sick: not just in the morning but for most of the day, and especially at night. The only thing that she could eat and keep down was Special K cereal. Everything that I ate completely nauseated her; I loved the coffee, the chocolate and, for the first time in my life, I'd discovered a love of meat. I didn't smoke, but everyone else in Spain did, and Nella used to retch walking down the street with me to fetch another packet of Special K. We didn't see as much of Spain as we'd planned to, but it was great to have a month in another place, and allowed us to get used to the idea of what was happening and to bond over it. I don't think that would have happened if we were in Australia running our usual lives. Then we came back home and told everyone the news. As soon as we arrived we morphed into a happy young couple expecting a baby. We started sharing our finances and became a team, ready to start a family.

Nella set up her own private dietetics practice in Byron Bay, designed to be a flexible part-time job that could be put into hibernation for the birth of our baby, and re-opened some months (or years) later when the time was right. A fast and furious six-month stint of preparation and work followed for her – right up until three days before the birth.

At the same time we desperately started searching for a place of our own to start building a nest during our second trimester. We found a small apartment in Mullumbimby, at the back of a house owned by our friends Ben and Shamila. (The same Ben who would later become the goalkeeper for our football team.) They had a young baby of six months, which was a great learning experience for us. Our families were good support for each other, even if ours hadn't quite yet got underway.

All this was way before I met Jim and he asked me to join the Rusty Trombones FC. That would be two years later, after April was born and we were expecting our second child.

The pregnancy books that Nella and I were reading at the time of this first pregnancy and birth were medical encyclopaedias full of all the horrible conditions and complaints that your baby could possibly suffer from. I stopped reading them because I was terrified. I knew things could and did happen, I just didn't want to know all the details about every single one of them. I wanted to put my best possible positive energy into this child. My rationale went something along the lines of: most children are born naturally and healthy – even in India, one of the most populous nations on earth where many people are without the access to modern technology that we have here – and ours will be too.

We attended a six-week course of pre-natal classes in Brunswick Heads. These were quite good and we made some new friends among the other couples expecting babies around the same time as us. Although we were planning a fairly non-medical birth at a local birthing centre, the classes gave us some useful information about what to expect before, during and after birth, including breastfeeding, changing cloth nappies, and so on. We also attended the standard eighteen-week scan, which checks if the baby is growing normally and looks for defects.

Our plan was to have the safest, in-control birth experience we could. We decided to use the best of both worlds: the modern medical technology and equipment of a hospital birthing centre, and the alternative ideals of pre-labour at home. We hired a wonderful doula called Penny for about $600 – a qualified midwife costs at least $2000. A doula is an experienced birth assistant with some training who has done coursework with a midwife or another doula. A midwife is certified and registered. Penny would be with us at all times as an advisor we knew and trusted so that our birth plan could be followed, be it at home or at the birthing centre.

We had always planned to do a lot of the pre-labour at home; we'd booked into the local birthing centre, but thought if we got there too early then they might ship us off to the hospital for intervention if the birth didn't progress quickly enough. A natural birth was something we both wanted. Well, I suppose Nella wanted it most; she was the one going through the ordeal after all, so whichever way she wanted to do it was the way I wanted to do it too. She was strong and very confident about her body – she'd always been fit, a triathlete even, was used to pushing her body and also relaxing it with yoga, so she was low-risk and hoped for a simple, natural birth.

She started having mild contractions at home while I was at work. I was shocked. It was ten days early and Nella's belly was still tiny; even Penny thought she had longer to go. She was in the middle of a cleaning frenzy, using her first day of maternity leave to scrub the floors on her hands and knees, which apparently is quite often the sign a woman is about to go into labour.

We were also midway through renovating the little flat, all the baby items were still packed away in boxes and Nella was frantically unpacking boxes and putting the baby clothes into the chest of drawers, which was still outside and freshly sanded back. She had to wait until I got home to move it inside the baby's room. I got the call at my office at about 2 p.m. and wanted to go straight home, a short ten-minute drive, but Nella insisted I get her two things: some Roy Orbison music (I didn't even know she liked Roy Orbison), and some of those lovely purple flowers growing on the street behind our house.

Thirty minutes later I arrived with my two gifts, only for her to say, 'I don't need that stuff now. I'm having a baby!' and then promptly vomit on the floor. There's no arguing with a woman in labour, let me tell you.

Nella laboured at home for what seemed like several hours. I called my mother and Carlie, Nella's friend, who would act as birth support – a trusted friend to attend the birth (research I read has shown that the more support a woman has in labour the fewer the complications). I also called our doula, Penny, all the while following Nella around as she moaned and bent over nearly every object in the house – the table, the bed, the TV – during each contraction.

The contractions were fast and intense from about 2 p.m. onwards, every two-and-a-half minutes and lasting up to one minute. This was definitely the real deal. At some point I ate dinner – a spinach and fetta pie that Carlie had brought over – and it was the most delicious meal of my life. I swear it was so full of flavour and incredibly tasty, probably helped along by all the surging hormones and emotions I was feeling.

Nella was doing really well. I could see it was painful but she was handling the pain with breathing exercises and moving around to different positions. This reassured me and I was pretty relaxed, doing whatever I could to help out; moving cushions around, holding her hair while she vomited, rubbing her back and helping her walk around and around and around.

Just that morning, Ben and I had set up a huge old cast-iron bathtub from my dad's house in the backyard, the same tub I bathed in as a three-year-old when we first arrived in Australia. After about four hours of labour, Penny asked Nella if she wanted to get into the bath, to change the scenery. Nella remembers thinking while in the bath, *This would be so lovely, having a hot bath in the backyard surrounded by trees and watching the sun go down … if I wasn't having a baby!*

After an hour, she had an urge to go to the toilet, but nothing would come out. Then her waters broke and Penny said it appeared as if Nella was trying to push the baby out, and if we wanted to go to the birthing centre, we had better get moving, now. Nella was in two minds, it would have been quite easy to stay and have the baby at home, but Penny wasn't a qualified midwife yet and Nella didn't want to put her in a difficult position. Months later we discovered that Penny had been to dozens of home births already and it wouldn't have been a big ask. Ah, well.

So we raced off to the birthing centre, Nella bent over the back seat of my old Mercedes station wagon. She was fully dilated when we arrived and April arrived twenty minutes later. Nella was leaning on a beanbag and I caught April's hot little body as she came out. She was a sticky, skinny little thing and I passed her up to Nella so they could have immediate skin-to-skin contact. As I passed her up the hospital midwife used some tubes to suck out some meconium from her nose and mouth. So after only about fifteen seconds she lay there on the outside of Nella's belly for the first time. After ten minutes, little April started nuzzling around and looking for the breast, and mother and baby had the first of many breastfeeding bonding sessions.

I thought it went very quickly, time seemed to stand still and go fast at the same time, was it really six hours already? Or just an hour or so that Nella had been in labour?

It was so mind-blowing that first day – the love I felt for this little baby that I helped to create. I had created life. I was so over the moon. It was far and away the best thing that had ever happened to me. Immediately, I felt this overwhelming sense of protection and love. Everything else fell away. Nothing could have happened that would have distracted me at that moment – an apocalypse outside the hospital wouldn't have bothered me.

It was a great start. And a good thing, because little April gave us hell for a year and a half with sleep deprivation. For the first three months she was your average baby at night, waking up every three hours for a breastfeed, but then she screamed through the entire day. Then, for the next fifteen months, she was your average happy baby during the day, and screamed through the entire night.

We left the birthing centre the day after April's birth and I remember thinking, What do we do with this thing now? Where is the advice? Where are the people who should be telling us what to do? It seemed unbelievable that we were thrown into this thing, this most important thing, with no training. I've never done this before. She screams. Is she hungry? Is she tired? We soon realised that we had been caught up in focusing largely on the birth. When the birth was going to happen. Having a good birth. What could go wrong with the birth. Then, once we actually had the baby, we were so relieved that the birth was over. But what we should have been focusing on was the fact that we would soon be responsible for a new human life that was totally dependent on us. We'd been building up to a six-hour birth for nine months and all of a sudden we had a baby life on our hands 24/7. It gave me a lot of respect for other parents. Everyone does it and everyone must feel this way the first time. We coped pretty well, I think, but early on I had the feeling that I wasn't qualified to do this.

We were given some support from a local early childhood centre. A midwife dropped in each day for a week after the birth, and offered us advice on breastfeeding, vaccinations and general support. To be honest we didn't find it that useful, and often got different messages from different staff regarding what would work for April. Penny, our doula, also dropped in several times after the birth and made sure we were doing okay.

The sleep deprivation that comes with young babies was a new experience for me. I'd been my own boss since age twenty and I'd never had to set an alarm; I simply woke up when I wanted and started work when I liked.

Now we were not sleeping for more than two hours at a time without April waking and screaming. After about six months, we went to a day-long course at a sleep school, where parents learn techniques to settle and get their babies to sleep through the night, or at least for more than one forty-minute sleep cycle.

We tried all the initiatives they suggested including controlled crying, a widely used sleep technique for managing infants and young children who do not settle alone or who wake at night. With controlled crying you leave the infant to cry for increasingly longer periods before providing comfort, which was really uncomfortable for us and against our instincts of 'love them so much they won't have anything to cry about', but we were going crazy with the lack of sleep and we were willing to try anything. Try we did, but it still didn't work. It was wearing us down and a few months later, with April now ten months, we went to a five-day 'baby boot camp' sleep-school intensive in Brisbane. We stayed overnight and were monitored closely – this helped a little for the first few days while staying there, but she was still up for a minimum of three hours a night screaming hysterically. Worse for us, if we stayed with her she screamed even more hysterically.

It broke my heart. We reached the stage where we just couldn't take it anymore – we even said to each other, and only slightly didn't mean it, 'You can understand how people can shake their children.' Sometimes Nella would be at breaking point and I'd calm her down and other times I'd be at breaking point and Nella would calm me down.

We did the full five days at sleep school and continued with their preferred method of controlled crying when we got home. It worked for about three weeks and then she reverted back to the screaming we knew so well. We would have to move *into* sleep school for this to work!

I started working from home to provide more support for Nella, but it was not a wise move as I only had a thin sheet separating my desk from our screaming child in her cot. Needless to say I didn't get as much work done as I hoped, but it was good to be in it together with Nella. We really suffered through it as a couple and I had a complete understanding of what full-time parenting meant. The noise just got into your head.

People would freely offer us advice: 'You should try aromatherapy', 'Why don't you try homeopathy?', 'You should use herbs', 'Craniosacral is excellent, and it worked for us.' We'd get a little annoyed, thinking, You have no idea what we've tried; we've tried everything. Literally everything available.

April was such a happy little person during the day with everyone she met, but at night, and when we tried to put her down for day sleeps, she screamed like a hysterical demon. Nella or I would hold her for hours at a time and she just would not calm down. My mother offered to take her for a night so we could get some decent rest, but she brought her back an hour later. She couldn't take it and was worried about the intensity of the screaming. She couldn't believe that's what we were putting up with all night, every night. It was such a big sound to come out of such a little person. I wanted to record it, just so I could play it back to people (and to April in years to come) – it was an unbelievable scream – but Nella felt too traumatised by it. So, after a year and a half of getting between three and five hours sleep a night – in forty-minute to two-hour-long snatches – we tried witchcraft.

It's not under W in the yellow pages, or even in the phone books of the alternative communities surrounding Nimbin and Byron Bay. But we heard from friends of friends of friends a story about a local woman who called herself a witch, who had exorcised a teenage spirit that was tormenting a young boy, so we gave her a call and left a message. Then I remembered that I'd read something about this in my early twenties when I was seeing a therapist/counsellor/mystic/witch (I'm sure that's not what it said on her business cards). I was dealing with bouts of depression at the time, and did a year of introspective self-analysis using a variety of mainstream and alternative personal-development techniques – I was having my mid-life crisis early.

So I read up on witchcraft again and that night, a Sunday, before we put April to bed, we burned a black candle in her room. We used a smudge stick (burning a bundle of dried herbs) and made clear intentions for bad energy to leave the room and the house. We poured a ring of salt around her cot to take up the bad energies. We put a symbol under her bed – something Nella was given by a friend – and we put piles of salt across the window frames and the door frame. We used a lot of salt. We had a couple of kilo bags of Saxa and made sure it covered every entrance and that there were no gaps. And while we're at it, we thought, why not hang a couple of garlic bulbs in her room as well – can't do any harm.

Then we put April to bed. And, do you know what? She slept through the entire night for the first time in her short life. It freaked us out. What had she been going through? Had something been tormenting her? It was a real turning point in her ability to sleep – she started sleeping through the night – and I can tell you, the world is a lot more beautiful when you get to sleep through the night.

The witch never returned our message, and didn't need to: maybe just the intention had helped. I didn't really believe in the witchcraft we'd tried – maybe I preferred not to open up a whole world I didn't know anything about, ignorance being bliss and all – but it had worked. About a year later we saw a naturopath for some help getting April to sleep (she still struggled with that) and he summed it up for us. 'Lots of things go through April,' he told us, 'she is like a super-sensitive radio, she picks up all signals, and can't turn down the volume.' The theory being that April tuned in to spirits, ghosts – whatever is out there – while she slept, and couldn't turn it off or down. These days, I can hardly hear the scream in my memory. April is four, a beautifully happy little girl who sleeps ... most of the night, most of the time.

It was around the time of the sleepless nights that I first met Jim and he asked me if I wanted to join a slapped-together soccer team. I knocked it back, as I did with many other things at that time; we were just so exhausted from the sleep deprivation. I think the weekly commitment also scared me off, as well as the idea of playing with a bunch of other guys who quite possibly could have been playing their whole lives (how little I knew) and would make me look and feel like an idiot.

We always wanted to have more than one child. We thought having a single child wouldn't be much fun for the lone little one growing up. And even though we'd had such a rough time, we knew that each child has a different personality and it was unlikely to be as hard the second time. Some couples we knew had a dream run the first time – a perfect baby – then had a second one and it was a screaming and non-sleeping nightmare, so we thought our chances were pretty good to have an easy one the next time. It couldn't get any harder, could it?

We'd had six months of getting our daily, and more importantly, nightly, lives back on track. April was now in family day care for two full days, and my mother was very keen to babysit a third day each week. My website business was flourishing in an office in Mullumbimby, my first apprentice had just graduated and I'd taken on a second apprentice. April was sleeping, we were working, socialising, playing tennis and surfing and we agreed that becoming pregnant anytime from now would be okay. We decided we wouldn't really try, we were in no hurry, but we'd stop using contraceptives, including the most reliable one – abstinence due to lack of sleep.

It had been nearly two years since April's birth, it was my thirtieth birthday and Nella had a surprise weekend planned for me. We went to Brisbane and April went happily to my mother's – which was a surprise. We stayed at a five-star hotel – which was a surprise. We went to a couple of fancy bars and restaurants – which was a surprise too. Then Nella told me that she was pregnant, which was the biggest surprise of all. We had fallen pregnant the first month. Another couple of months of our more relaxed lifestyle would have been nice, but I was very happy. We also worked out this baby would probably be a Libran which we hoped would make them calmer than our highly strung, yet beautiful, Aries girl, April.

Nella was sick again during the second pregnancy, although not as badly as the first time. While it was easier in some ways – like anything you do more than once – it was harder in other ways because it was compounded by the fact that there was already one child running around, eating, pooing, sleeping (sometimes), demanding (at all times), scribbling on the walls and climbing on the chairs. You can't just lie down when you feel a bit tired or ill. And I was working. It was different from the first time around, it wasn't: 'We're going to have a baby – wow!' We were trying to run an already full life. We'd just come out of the tunnel of a year and a half of no sleep and we were about to go back in again for at least another six months (best case scenario). Plus we'd just started getting our sex life back in order, and becoming pregnant the first month ran the sex train right off track, through the tunnel of no sleep and into a barren ditch beyond it.

I think for many women the lack of sex is not a big deal, but for me, as for most men, it was because sex was a big part of my connection with my partner. I love her, and sex is how I feel that deep bond and intimacy with her. Without sex it's like being just good friends. I've had relationships like that and didn't want this one to become 'just' a friendship, however good that friendship was. So the pregnancy was tough.

We decided I needed to work to allow Nella time at home – better the mum at home, we thought. She gave away her private practice as a dietician and I became the sole provider again. If I could provide financially for Nella, April and a new baby, I was happy for her to stay at home with the kids until they went to school. Coming home from work after a full day, tired and weary (and not having sex), does sometimes feel like a thankless task, but it was easier to accept the second time around as we knew what it was going to be like and we could both see the bigger picture. And also every tiny smile in the morning made it all worthwhile.

We didn't attend classes and I didn't read any books to prepare for the second pregnancy. We didn't want any scans, and didn't want to know the sex of the baby. We knew Jim was panicking about their pregnancy and having a healthy baby, but we were happy not to know and to deal with things as they came up.

Jim asked me again to join the football team, now called Fertile FC because all the players' partners were pregnant. I'd been to see a few games in season one, realised how basic most of their football skills were, how un-seriously they took it, and how much fun they were having. I'd also met Nick, Neil and Ross briefly at social gatherings at Jim's house and on a surfing trip, and this made me feel more comfortable about joining the group. Team sports weren't big in the commune I grew up in, so I've never been very sporty. Nella encouraged me, thinking it would be good for me to hang out with more men and get fitter, to balance the sedentary nature of computer work. So every Thursday I was able to get away from the family and spend some time kicking and screaming on a soccer field with other men who were all in the same situation of either having young children or just about to become fathers.

We decided that we would have a home birth, as the previous birth would've been one if we hadn't left for the birthing centre when we did. There was no extra technology or apparatus at the birthing centre that we couldn't have at home. If intervention was needed, then Nella would be taken in an ambulance to a hospital up the coast. By now we had moved out of our tiny flat into a large, ramshackle farmhouse on sixty acres, an ideal setting, so we thought we might as well be at home.

Once that was decided, we found an experienced registered midwife who was happy to oversee a home birth and agreed on a fee. This included meeting us for four to six weeks beforehand, attending the birth and following up at our home afterwards. The laws regarding midwifery insurance have changed since, and now anyone attending a home birth must have adequate, and expensive, insurance. We couldn't afford to pay her until we got the federal government's baby bonus after the birth, but she was happy to wait. She had a lot of experience with home births and said that, statistically, there were far fewer complications and interventions at home births due mainly to the fact that the mother was relaxed. She had all the apparatus and knowledge and was backed up by another midwife who was on call if for any reason our midwife was unavailable at a crucial time.

Nella wanted a water birth this time around. We had heard it was more comfortable to labour in water, to be weightless and move around easily into any position that felt comfortable. It also took some of the physical pressure off Nella's body – God knows, there was enough pressure with the baby bearing down – and the transition for the baby from the amniotic fluid into water would be much smoother. This was apparently less stressful for the baby, since it had floated in fluids for the first nine months. We'd wanted a water birth the first time around too but, as it took forty minutes to fill the bath at the birthing centre and Nella had the baby only twenty minutes after arriving, a puddle birth was all that would have been possible.

So this time a birthing pool was delivered to our home a few weeks before the due date by our midwife. It is an inflatable pool specially designed for birthing, with reinforced walls and handles in appropriate places for squeezing until white-knuckled. We were relaxed about the birth, we knew it had taken six hours the first time, so we started to inflate the pool in the living room when Nella started to have early contractions and began her labour.

That night, Nella couldn't sleep. She whispered to me in bed, 'I think we're going to have our baby tonight.' Nella didn't want me to phone anyone, but I said, 'Nella, you're having a baby, you're going to have to inconvenience some people.' I phoned my mother, who came within ten minutes. The plan was that if April woke up and freaked out, then Mum was going to take her to her place, but if she didn't they were going to stay. I also phoned Carlie. She arrived after thirty minutes. Carlie was one of Nella's best friends and had been support person for April's birth too. By this time she was training to be a nurse and midwife. Finally

I phoned the midwife – she had done around 250 births so we felt more comfortable with her as a birth specialist than a doctor. We were confident we could do this, but we wanted the midwife there as well, of course.

Once the pool was inflated and full of warm water, Nella began walking about and felt it was happening pretty quickly. I phoned the midwife again after about half an hour and told her, 'It's not just pre-labour, the contractions are intense and two minutes apart.' Half an hour later, however, the midwife still wasn't there and I called her again, 'Okay, I'll be there in twenty minutes,' she said. By now, Nella was in the pool, moaning with the contractions. She was leaning over the side of the pool and I was supporting her physically and emotionally. It was obviously close, we could feel the head. Thirty minutes later, just as I was getting ready to call her again, the midwife walked through the door. Right then Nella's waters broke, she felt as if she could push and ten minutes later our second baby was born.

I was holding Nella so I couldn't catch the baby this time. We asked Carlie if she wanted to do it, her first, and she gladly said, 'Can I?' With a water birth the baby doesn't take its first breath until they come up from underwater. This meant we needed to make sure the baby didn't break the surface, breathe and then go back under – which the midwife took control of – so Carlie caught the baby when it came. As Nella lay in the pool with our new baby, I stripped off and jumped in too – much like an instinctive skinny-dip at a great pool party – except in this case the pool only just had room for two adults and a small baby.

It was very much the same feeling as with April's birth. I had some fear that I wouldn't think it was as life-changing and momentous as the first time. But it was. Straight back to that zone, many of the same feelings. We didn't even look to see if it was a boy or a girl immediately. We had never thought about a gender preference during the pregnancy. The midwife asked and we looked – a baby boy. We had a mattress laid out nearby, pulled out a doona, cleaned the baby up and lay down with him. The midwife wasn't doing very much at all actually, but we'd agreed that she would be in the background, there to answer questions, but not intervene unless we requested or needed it. I cut the cord and the midwife dissected the placenta. It was quite incredible to see the patterns and colours of the placenta, all those veins and membranes that fed our little boy for his first nine months. I wasn't sure at the time that I wanted to see it but it was really worthwhile. The midwife told us how you can tell how healthy the baby was, and how well the pregnancy had gone, by looking inside the placenta. For instance, the placenta of a smoker's baby can be a different colour and a third of the size of a healthy baby's placenta. Placentas can pump for hours afterwards and they're often left attached for some time. We felt very safe and supported having our very own midwife on hand; it was definitely worth the money we paid to have this great experience.

Little man, what shall we call you? Nella liked Sonny. I liked Frankie. But we waited for a few days and tried a different name each day to see which fitted best. I didn't think Frankie suited. Sonny worked well as he had a head of glowing, golden hair. So Sonny it was, and I could pick the middle name. Marcel was an old school friend from Nimbin who I'd been close to when we were younger. He died tragically in a car accident just a year earlier so I was happy to remember him and name my son Sonny Marcel.

It was lovely. We were home. It had been a two-and-a-half hour labour. No visiting hours – anyone could come and no one had to leave. We sat around with cups of tea talking and grinning until about 4 a.m., when Mum and Carlie went off to have a sleep and we went to bed.

April, at two and a half, slept through the whole thing and when she woke the next morning there was one extra person in the house. She came running in to us at seven o'clock and jumped into our makeshift bed to see him. We had explained the pregnancy and birthing process to her and she understood what was going on. We had told her, 'Mummy might be making lots of sounds and be in some pain, but it's okay, she did that with you too.' There was no jealousy, April was very gentle with the new baby and loved holding him straight away. We'd done some preparation with her, making sure she felt a part of it – when people came round in those first few days they were to ask April if she could show them her baby brother, which she was delighted to do. 'I've got a baby brother,' she would tell them. Later on she would occasionally say to me, 'Dad, I don't want to be a big sister anymore, it's too hard.' Because she had to be patient, couldn't snatch toys away or push him around in a trolley when he didn't like it – and it was hard for her, but she was learning to be a great big sister.

I didn't think I'd be able to love the second baby enough. I'd given all my love to the first baby, how could I love any more? But you do. It's extra love. You have more love there, inside of you somewhere. There's no rationing of love. It's a silly thing to fear perhaps and maybe it's not so instantaneous with subsequent children but the love thing definitely happens wholly for each child. You never really get the opportunity to just look and stare and wonder at the second baby as much, though, because you're bathing, feeding, working, sleeping and caring for two. I probably looked in wonder at April a lot more.

Then it all started again – the bathing, the feeding, the changing, the settling and the snatching sleep whenever we could – and now all times two. Nella breastfed Sonny and he was a real guzzler; no problems at all with the feeding. I had three weeks off work and went out infrequently, usually to play football with my new mates.

The first three games I was so sore I couldn't walk for two days after. Every muscle in my legs hurt, and only when Neil passed on his tip about bathing in Epsom salts after the game did the sore legs stop. Another enduring memory I have of my first games playing football is being so nervous I couldn't kick the ball more than five metres. Each Thursday I would have butterflies in my stomach and could barely eat from the anxiety and excitement about that night's game. Pre-game and warm up were okay, but once on the pitch I was a mess of nerves and pretty useless. I didn't score a goal that season, but I did feel that some sense of ability was starting to show itself and I was having a great time bonding with my team mates – united in our inability to play 'the beautiful game'. I also loved learning the technical side of football, the awareness of where everyone in the team needs to be, that each person plays a crucial role, not just the goalie and striker. I was learning more each game and applying it to the next.

Staying for a quick sideline beer after a game was great. Reliving the glorious moments and laughing about the disastrous ones. In one game we played an A-grade team, the 'Pirates', and we figured if we lost less than 10–0 to them we'd count it as a win. By the end of the game it was 9–1 to them and we celebrated like we'd won. I don't think the Pirates knew what to make of us.

I remember once, after only a week or so, trying to sound like a pro (professional father, not footballer): 'Anyone going for a beer after the game?' I asked. 'I don't have to head off straight away. I can stay for a beer or two.' The rest of the team looked at me with quiet, blokey admiration. They hadn't given birth yet, and saw it as a triumph of manhood that one could stay out for a beer within only a few weeks of having a new baby. Ten minutes later, on the way to the bar I got the call. 'Yes, okay, of course, straight away, I'll be there in ten minutes,' and immediately and rather sheepishly had to leave to go home. What was I thinking?

For the next few weeks Nella and I lived and breathed the new two-child family life. As you can imagine, there's a lot of cooperation and a lot of juggling required. We had to be a good team – to be strong together – and it's probably strengthened our relationship. If we did resort to emotional blackmail, we didn't take it personally – we both knew it was the fatigue talking. When you have a child together, your relationship definitely takes a back seat, but you have to try to consider each other while you're both in the back seat. You learn to say sorry, and learn to say it quicker so the issue is resolved and you can both move on.

Being a father already, I was really looking forward to the other men in the team becoming fathers (and hoping it wouldn't be as hard for them as it was for me). I didn't want to tell them what it was like for me, or taint them with my experiences, not until after they had their own birth experience and kids, then we could talk about it. Like seeing a movie, I'd rather discuss it with people who have already seen it, not those who are about to see it.

Three weeks after Sonny's birth, I started going to work early in the morning. When I came home from work at

5.30 p.m., I'd walk in the door and straight away I'd be bathing, feeding or putting kids to bed – sometimes still with my shoes and jacket on and my bag over my shoulder. I'd take them to bed, read a story, have a cuddle and put them to sleep. By this point it would be 8.30, I'd have something to eat and I'd be wrecked and ready for bed. Ready to do it all again the next day.

I took Fridays off work for the rest of the year, which was a blessing for the family but not for the business. So I started working at night after the kids went to bed. Nella would go to bed at 8.30 then I'd spend another three or so hours on the laptop. It was stressful at times, but mostly I just knew what I had to do for my family, and I did that matter-of-factly.

Like his big sister, Sonny never really started sleeping through the night. He'd wake at one, at three, at four and at five. I'd share settling him and then I'd have to go to work. The number of times I had only four hours sleep (one or two hours at a time) was way too many. I often thought, How the hell am I going to get through the day? I'd have meetings where I'd have to impress clients with my business and look at them through eyes that hurt with fatigue. But you get through it. However little sleep we got with Sonny, we always remembered how much worse it had been with April.

There were times when I wanted Nella to know how hard my day had been. I'd come home and she would say how difficult the kids had been: Sonny didn't want to eat lunch, April had almost swallowed a battery, etc. For my part, I hadn't even been to the toilet all day, hadn't had lunch, hadn't stopped for one minute. I'd had six people wanting something from me every second, the phone ringing, meetings planned, the phone ringing, staff to be paid, clients who hadn't paid, projects that were behind, the phone ringing. I'd have a massive day and then get home and it all starts. Sometimes I wanted Nella to know that I'd also been working very hard. Not to belittle her day and how hard she'd been working, but so she'd appreciate my situation too. But often there was no time to talk until the kids were in bed. We'd try to eat together, but if the kids were having trouble going to sleep, we'd take it in turns to eat dinner and look out for them. We did try to get at least half an hour to talk every day, but by then we were completely exhausted and the half-hour was probably best spent sleeping.

There are a lot of really good things about having a baby. Becoming much more selfless and realising that I have a higher purpose than just fulfilling my own little wants, needs and desires is a major one. I feel like I'm actually creating something, I'm responsible for something and it's not about me and I'm okay with that, okay with being part of something bigger. Another thing is passing on your legacy. Showing your children what you believe is the right way to live and how to treat other people. I'll bring kids up to do the right thing and respect other people and that'll make the world a better place. I'm happy I'm passing on my own values, morals and ethics, just like my father did for me.

We all do the best we can and hopefully it gets better and better. As a child I had plenty of freedom, whereas Nella had a stricter upbringing. I think our children will have a nice balance of the two. We give them respect but expect respect in return. We let them learn their own lessons. We will tell April and Sonny if the fire is hot, or the tea is hot, or the food is spicy, but only once and if they don't listen then they can learn that lesson themselves. And they do learn – to trust their own judgement, to listen, and to be heard as well, their opinion is just as important as ours. We do set some ground rules and boundaries, such as no hitting, teasing or jumping off cliffs, but in general our kids are very easy to get along with, they are respectful of other people's belongings and we can trust them to do as we ask.

Having children is the best thing I've ever done in my life. But on the other hand, it's the hardest thing I've ever done, too. It's challenging in so many ways – like giving up my life and lifestyle. Having children, you really get to appreciate any time on your own – just to listen to your favourite music, or enjoy some precious silence.

When we're not training or playing in the six-a-side comp, I play a casual Sunday football game in Mullumbimby. Anyone who turns up can play and it's great fun, good for fitness and meeting new people. Some Sundays when Nella can't mind the kids I bring them along, carting down the picnic rug, toys, water bottles, food and blankets to keep them happy. If they are happy, I can play football, and I'm happy. I'll jog back every five minutes for a drink of water and to check on them, they love it and act like my personal bar staff, 'More water, Daddy?', 'Yummy nuts, Daddy?' April, being a true little princess, sometimes looks like a big ball of pink fluff sitting on the sidelines, with her pink blanket, pink toys, pink ballerina dress, pink shoes and happy pink face. Sometimes Rick and Ross join me and we make sure we play on the same team, practising our passing with each other, little triangles, Rick doing his deadly runs up the left wing, passing to me in the centre, and then I slip it through to Ross waiting in the goal box, ever the sharpshooter.

The one thing I'd say to someone who is contemplating having a child is, 'You can do it.' You'll do it your own way – and I don't have any extraordinary advice that will make you a better father – but you are capable of doing it. Everyone is, that's the great thing. Whatever your background, you can be a good parent and kids make you do that. Everyone has their doubts, of course. Can I love a child? Then, can I love my second child as much? It's truly one of the most beautiful things to see your two kids talking to each other and having their own relationship together. It's an incredible ride and you can do it if you want to.

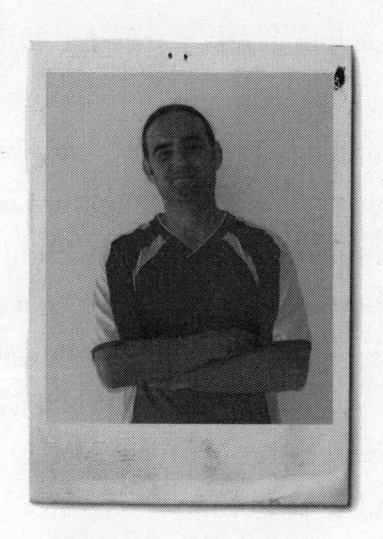

ROSS' STORY

A right-footed attacker who can take men on and will score goals. He plays fair but hard and doesn't give up the chase easily. He grew up playing football in the Scottish streets and parks of Glasgow and is not unfamiliar with the physical side of the game. Ross can turn and spin round his marker in a flash and uses the ball well. He also uses his hands a lot when speaking, an attribute that contributes to his skills as an unyielding goalkeeper when called upon.

IT'S NOT LIKE I HAD A PLAN — I MEAN, NOT A PLAN I WAS

aware of – just lots of little plans that sort of got stuck on the end of each other and pushed me along my journey in life. I grew up in Glasgow, Scotland. Glasgow had and maybe still does have (courtesy of Billy Connolly and *Taggart*) a reputation as being a hard, gritty city, although the shipyards now lie quiet and heavy industry is shrinking. I was a seventies' baby growing up in the Thatcher years of the eighties – privatisation, coal strikes, high unemployment and weirdly tight football shorts.

As a young boy, football was everything. At school we played at every break and lunchtime and kicked a ball between us on the walk home. In Glasgow there were two main football teams: Celtic and Rangers. If you were Catholic you supported Celtic, and if you were Protestant you supported Rangers. This wasn't always the case, and my parents never forced it on me, but culturally there was never any real choice. I was born a Catholic and so it was a green and white hooped football strip for me. I played in the school football team and loved it – even in snow, when we had to use an orange ball. I played for quite a few years until my pals and I started getting into skateboarding and decided that it was more fun terrorising shoppers as we jumped down stairs in the local shopping centre car park.

I was the eldest of three boys, each of us two years apart. We played together in the street as I grew up, but as I got older I was out with friends a lot more than I was home. This was the start of what my mum referred to as my years of 'burning the candle at both ends'. It was a life of girls, dance parties, cheap booze, hanging out in parks and train stations and doing some work to get the cash to pay for it all. I was accepted into university and continued to have a good time and work a range of jobs for cash to finance the fun.

I had been working in a Pizza Hut delivery shop for a while and one day a pretty girl came in and handed over a job application while I was standing out front with my manager. As she walked out, he turned to me and said, 'What do you think?', and with no hesitation I said, 'Yeah!' and she was in. Little did I know at that point who that pretty girl was to become in my life.

The pretty girl, Bella, soon became my girlfriend. She was doing a design degree at the Glasgow School of Art and we had lots in common. However, I had already made a decision to do some overseas voluntary work. Over the phone I thought they had said Tasmania, which seemed a bit weird but I went along with it, and found out later it was actually Tanzania – just a bit different. Bella helped me fundraise and was very supportive even though she was really sad to see me go away for three months. By that point she had taken time off from her studies and had decided she was going to go to Asia and Australia. She suggested that we could travel together when I got back from Africa. Sounded good to me – certainly put off having to make any decisions about the future for a while – so we had a plan, the first of many Bella and I were to have together.

I spent three months in rural Tanzania, living in a tent, making bricks and building a health centre while talking basic Swahili with the locals. I didn't have much with me, but I did have one thing – a football. The universal language of football made me so many friends and I spent every dusty evening kicking the ball around the pitch with the kids and the older guys. We even organised a game: our village against another village an hour's walk away – our team were 'skins' and my skinny white top half was of much amusement to the local girls.

Once back with Bella in Glasgow, we packed up, said goodbye to our parents and set off on what was to be our big adventure.

After travelling through Asia, we ended up working on a remote Aboriginal community in the Great Victoria Desert for six months – and this was where I watched the 1998 World Cup. It was also there that we fell hook, line and sinker in love with Australia, and dreamed of the possibility of one day living in this awesome place.

We returned to Glasgow with heavy hearts, but five years later another few plans had come off and we were off on another adventure – a new beginning. Soon we were on a plane back to Australia, permanent resident visas in the passports, a first-class honours degree and post-grad certificate in the bag, and wedding rings on our fingers.

We had a whole country to choose from – where to live? A map sat on the floor of our Glasgow living room for months. We had loved Byron Bay, so the plan was to live in a kombi and see if we could get jobs and make it work there. Soon enough we were both in full-time professional employment and living in Mullumbimby – the biggest little town in Australia – which we had fallen in love with for its eclectic mix of drop-out hippies, socially aware professionals and traditional farming conservatives.

I met Neil while working at Uncle and I met Jim through him. Jim and I had a few skate sessions and Neil and I had many, many drinking sessions. When Jim suggested the Summer Sixes soccer comp I was well up for it. Apart from occasional skateboarding and some body-surfing, I was getting unfit and my flat stomach was a thing of the past. Bella was supportive and even envious that I had this excuse for fun and fitness. The first season was brilliant – we totally went for it (on the pitch and off). The games were hard, and after winning the first game easily we had a much harder job for the next nine weeks. During a game mid-season, I committed to a 50/50 ball, I made it but he did too – just a second later. I knew it was bad straight away, my toe was agony. I tried to play on but came off for a rest a few minutes later. I played most of the second half and went back to Jim's as usual before going home.

That night, I woke up at 3 a.m. in unbelievable pain. The next day the doctor said I had broken my toe. He asked if I had stopped straight away to put ice on it, and I said, 'Yes, of course' – I had rested my cold bottle of beer against it at Jim's house between sips. The next two games I played in goal before playing the last few with very strong painkillers in my system. It was really sore for months afterwards but I didn't want to miss any of the games.

At the after-match sessions, there were times when we laughed so much we cried. There were several characters in the team and their tales had us all in stitches. I can remember Rick telling an unforgettable story (which I've since forgotten) and I just couldn't believe the way he told it, everyone was holding their sides with laughter and he just kept going – deadpan – it was hilarious. They were a good bunch of lads who knew how to have fun but who also knew how to go to work the next day and be considerate to others. The football to some extent was secondary. I only knew a couple of them at the start of the ten-week season, but by the end of it we were all pretty close and we started hanging out a lot more.

Bella and I had now been together for twelve years and had never given the idea of having children much thought – not because we didn't want children, we just hadn't come to the point where we really did. I can't remember having any babies around when I was growing up – there probably were but I was out playing football all the time. I had held the daughter of one of my best mates when she was a baby, but I was always so nervous, as if I might break her, and was always scared that I would make her cry.

We had some fabulous years of being grown-ups with disposable incomes – working hard, partying with childless friends and going on holidays to child-free destinations. But after a few years we realised that while we loved our life, we had been doing the same thing for a while and we both felt it was the right time to move on to the next stage. I was thirty-two and Bella was thirty-one.

It was Bella who mentioned having a baby first, around October, and much to her surprise I agreed. It just felt right – if we were going to do it, why not now? What were we waiting for?

Bella is really into doing things the right way, which makes for a good balance in our relationship. She started doing some research and taking a vitamin formula that was supposed to help with healthy conception and pregnancy. I, on the other hand, was playing football to get fit but the after-game refreshments probably weren't helping. We decided to enjoy the excesses of one last cocktail-fuelled Christmas and New Year with our child-free friends, detox in January, and then start to try to have a baby.

We had a party at our place for Hogmanay (Scottish for New Year's Eve) and Jim and Sarah popped in. They told us their news that night – which was a big surprise and we were stoked for them, and also excited that we would at least know one other couple who would be going through the same stuff as we (hopefully) would be going through soon. I guess this was a big thing for us – being a long way from family and our old circle of friends, we felt a bit isolated. Our decision to try to start a family had been made with the realisation that we would not have the same support circle around us in Australia as we would have had if we were still in Glasgow.

So it was a case of 'Happy New Year, body, I'm going to start taking care of you now – for the first time in a long time.' Bella was now eating only organic food and doing lots of research into getting and being pregnant. It was a different place to be, a real shift from our normal lives up until then. I was a bit excited, a bit nervous, and a bit 'Oh shit, this is something I know absolutely nothing about.'

We were going to wait until February, but late in January we stopped using condoms. We had sex for the first time without a condom, then a few more times in quick succession. Sometimes there'd be demand for even more, as Bella had read approximately a million websites about it and explained to me how difficult it was to actually get pregnant. Well, we didn't want to fail at it, so we tried really, really hard! We had read about techniques that apparently give the best chance of getting pregnant – such as if the woman has an orgasm just after the man then it helps 'scoop in the sperm', helping it on its journey towards the egg – so we tried them all. One night in an attempt to get some mood lighting, I turned a wall lamp around so it glowed warmly up the purple wall. We were having sex and I could smell something burning – the lamp I'd turned around was burning a hole in the plasterboard wall of our newly renovated bedroom. It was at this time that Bella thinks we conceived, and although there is a picture over the hole now, it will always be there to remind us of that moment.

We were obviously hoping to get pregnant, but didn't really expect it to happen in the first week. I'd not been taking great care of my body for quite a few years and didn't know if my sperm were up to it. Bella felt she knew the day after the burning plasterboard, she told me she felt different and that last night may have done it. I was dubious, but went along with it. Bella wanted to take a pregnancy test about a week after the burning-hot-love night. I'd just been for my annual skin cancer test and they had taken a specimen away for testing. Now that I was trying to have a child, it brought up the issue of my own mortality and I didn't want to find out that Bella was pregnant while I was waiting to hear if I had cancer. I told Bella of my concerns but she was too excited and too used to my unfounded anxieties. She says I have 'man flu tendencies', whatever that means.

She had bought a pregnancy kit, but had agreed with me not to use it yet. Then she secretly got up at five o'clock the next morning and did the test. She looked at it and the 'you're pregnant' second line came up straight away, but was so faint that you couldn't really see it. Despite me not wanting her to do the test, Bella couldn't keep it to herself that she had done it and was unsure of the result. So we did another test again after work and got the same result

– a faint second line. We were confused. So Bella phoned the helpline on the pregnancy kit and asked them about the faint line, and they were definite that a second line, however faint, meant pregnant. Bella explained that it was really, *really* faint, but they were adamant that any sign of a line meant she was pregnant, and that it would just be faint because it was so early in the pregnancy.

Despite their certainty, Bella felt she needed clarification from a doctor before she could be sure, so went to see one in her lunch hour the next day. She requested a blood test, but the doctor would only do another pee test. When the result came back, he confidently said, 'You are definitely not pregnant.' Bella was a bit shocked and again asked if she could have a blood test, but the doctor told her not to worry, that she was young and could try again. She showed him the two other tests she had done and explained that the manufacturer's helpline had assured her that any second line meant she was pregnant, but the doctor said, 'Well, they can't see the test. I can, and I am telling you that you are not pregnant.' Bella, being fairly strong-willed and feeling that she knew her own body, insisted on the blood test and he reluctantly agreed.

The next day, she phoned the nurse for the results, who confirmed that Bella was indeed pregnant. It wasn't until three days later that the doctor himself phoned and told Bella the result officially. When Bella said to him, 'You told me I wasn't pregnant', he replied that it wasn't him who had said she wasn't pregnant, it was the test. Bella was just glad she was so sure of her own body and that she had insisted on the blood test. If she had been a younger, less confident girl she could easily have taken the doctor's word for it and potentially gone out drinking, smoking, taking drugs and risked the pregnancy and the baby. Needless to say, we never went back to that doctor.

So there you go – it ended up being only a couple of weeks between having unprotected sex for the first time together and finding out we were pregnant. The downside was that as soon as we found out we didn't have sex every day any more.

You can think about becoming a dad and how it might feel, but as soon as you find out, life changes somehow. It was time for me to do different things in my life and I was happy and excited about that. Bella and I had a new plan and had started another new adventure together.

We agreed we shouldn't tell anyone for the first three months until the chances of a miscarriage were greatly reduced. The only people we told were Bella's sister, Louisa, who was in the country at the time, and Neil and Mette. It's a strange time as you have the biggest news of your life but you can't tell anyone – you walk around all day feeling totally different and wondering if anyone notices.

In March, Jim organised a surf trip to Angourie National Park with a group of guys including Yari, Nick, Neil and a few more surfers who I didn't really know. I was well up for a boys' camping trip but well out of my depth with the surfing. Around the fire one night, Jim was talking about how it felt to have a pregnant partner and we all listened intently. Then Yari piped up and announced he was also expecting a baby but was in the 'don't tell anyone' period. We all congratulated him, thanked him for sharing and promised we wouldn't tell anyone else. It turned out that Yari and Nella's baby was due on the same day as ours. What was I to do? We were in the 'don't tell anyone' time too, but so was Yari, and he'd shared. I was so keen to tell my mates but we'd promised not to tell anyone (else), so I didn't. Neil knew, and when the rest of the boys were all out surfing the big waves and we were nursing our big hangovers we had time to chat. It was good to have the time and space to have those conversations – we were all in the middle of a big life-changing experience and just talking about it out loud was important.

During the first trimester I tried to do what I could to help Bella, even though it was completely new ground for both of us. Bella was mega-tired, with some mild nausea, but she was lucky to escape without any morning sickness. It's a strange time in those first three months as you're excited about being pregnant but feel like you can't be too joyful until you pass that magic twelve-week mark. It was like the first part of the plan was done but that just opened up a whole Pandora's box of other things to worry about. I remember thinking that too much knowledge was a bit dangerous – being blissfully unaware of any possible complications would have been a good way to go. Despite the fact she was exhausted, and out of the house for twelve hours a day working at the same place as me on the Gold Coast, Bella was somehow finding time to do a lot of research and was constantly asking me questions about what I thought of things such as immunisations, dummies, the baby sleeping in the same bed with us, nappies, watching TV with the baby – all things I'd never even considered having an opinion about until then.

As the first trimester progressed, I was looking after Bella and starting to take a bigger share of cooking and cleaning duties. She was eating only organic foods and avoiding anything that wasn't good for the baby. This was also a big change for us – we were not mad keen on cooking; we cooked to eat, the quicker (and with the least washing up) the better. Now we were peeling vegetables, baking things and doing kitchen 'stuff' which we found we were ill-equipped – in skills and tools – to do, but again this was an essential learning experience for the adventure we were about to go on.

I was not reading anywhere near the amount Bella was, but enjoyed reading about the different stages the baby was going through: 'after two weeks, this and that'; 'after four weeks this and that'. At some stage I read that my son or daughter had a little tail – cool! Bella would tell me the highlights of all the reading and researching she'd been doing too – mostly on the hour drive to and from work. We decided early in the pregnancy that we wanted the birth to be as natural as possible. I agreed we should skip the twelve-week scan as Bella had read that there are associated risks for the foetus, and we had already decided that we wouldn't terminate the pregnancy if it came up with any abnormalities anyway.

Telling our parents over the telephone after the regulation three months was weird; it seemed the type of thing that you should do in person, but there was no chance of that. They were really excited and happy but their reaction was also tinged with sadness because the distance between us suddenly became even greater.

In the second trimester the tiredness subsided, and Bella felt great and loved being pregnant. Ideas and choices about parenting style – mostly on the natural side of the fence – were discussed. Bella was adamant that we make sure there was minimal opportunity for our baby to come into contact with toxins and wanted to have only natural, non-chemically treated products. Her research unearthed a scary number of baby products that were packed full of dangerous toxins, such as PVC change-mats, foam cot mattresses, and BPA-ridden teething toys and baby bottles. It was unbelievable that these things are allowed to be manufactured and given to our babies and children. Thankfully, some items, like baby bottles containing BPA, are now slowly being removed from the shelves by some companies. It just goes to show that what some people refer to as 'hippy alternatives' are actually more a matter of common sense. I know I sat up and took notice – I had a precious wee baby in there and I was going to do everything I could to protect it from anything harmful.

We had our first scan at eighteen weeks, just before we flew to Malaysia to have our last holiday as a couple – our 'babymoon'. Bella wanted to know if it was a boy or a girl. She had no real preference, but wanted a girl slightly more than a boy and wanted some time to get her head around it if it did turn out to be a boy. I'd always thought I'd want a boy to play football with and have adventures with. I grew up with two brothers and that's what I knew and felt more comfortable with – what would I do with a girl? But the more I thought about it, the more I realised I could do all that stuff, and more, with a daughter. The scan was weird and exciting; we saw our baby for the first time – even though it looked a bit like an alien. Unfortunately, the radiologist was less than impressed with our desire to know the baby's sex, telling us it was too hard to see and making no attempt to really try – so we left with it still a mystery.

We had a great holiday in Malaysia, lazing around, snorkelling and sightseeing. The evenings were a bit different from past holidays though, as after dinner Bella was ready for bed, so I would enjoy a few beers on the balcony with my book for company.

We were past the halfway mark now pregnancy-wise and some casual training sessions were happening football-wise. By this point, Yari, Rick, Neil and I were on the way to being fathers and Jim and Sarah had welcomed Bijou into the world – almost a whole six-a-side football team of good friends were about to go through this experience at the same time, which I was stoked about. We were bonding again, but in a deeper way. During the first season all our talk revolved around the past: funny stories that made us who we were. Now it was talk about the future: our worries, questions, advice and reassurance.

It was great that all my close friends were changing their lives and lifestyles at the same time. Rather than us all going out together with our partners to pubs, concerts and restaurants, we would be going out on adventures with our kids together – that sat really well with me.

Bella and I were still both working on the Gold Coast, and the travelling was a necessary evil. Bella had to use a computer a lot for work and developed sore wrists from what we thought was typing, like a repetitive strain injury. But after going to the doctor we found out it was carpal tunnel syndrome and was common in pregnant women during their second and third trimesters. She had constant pain and tingling in her arms and had to wear splints on her wrists to alleviate the symptoms. It's one of those things that can happen during pregnancy that you don't know about until you're actually pregnant. It was difficult for Bella to sleep with the pain in her hands and arms, as she had to keep her fingers and wrists moving to stop the cramps. Wearing the splints definitely helped, but she could really only wear one at a time as they limited her movement. She found it hard, but she was also pretty relieved that that was the only 'downside' of being pregnant that she'd experienced. Bella was also having weekly sessions with an acupuncturist who specialised in pregnancy. She started going because she suffers badly from hayfever and allergies, and despite the doctor's insistence that it was safe to take antihistamines while pregnant, Bella didn't want to. The acupuncture sessions worked a treat and greatly relieved her stuffy nose and watery eyes and the bonus was that the acupuncturist also helped with the carpal tunnel and regularly checked on the baby's progress.

In the second trimester we started to get more organised at home. There was one room that we hadn't renovated; it was to become the nursery and we had some work to do to turn it into a room fit for a new baby. That was my weekends sorted until the baby was born. I felt this was a good way for me to contribute while Bella did all the baby-growing hard work.

As the third trimester approached, Bella really wanted to know whether it was a boy or a girl. I was cool with finding out on the big day, but if Bella was going to find out there would be fat chance of me not knowing. So at thirty-three weeks we drove up to a clinic near Brisbane that had a 3D scanner. It was a mad experience, really different from the rural place where we had the first scan. The room they took us into had a big plush padded bed surrounded by La-Z-Boy recliners all facing a big screen on the wall. Mood lighting was set and the radiographer introduced herself and told us about the procedure. We explained that we wanted to know the sex and as soon as she started the scan she said, 'Congratulations, it's a boy.' 'A boy!' we said, looking at each other. 'No … no,' the radiographer said, almost straight away, 'it's a girl – it was just the cord I saw there.'

'Okay, so is it a girl or a boy?' I said.

'It's a girl … I'm ninety per cent sure – she has just moved round – I can't see any more.'

We had just been told the sex of our baby, or had we? We didn't know. The radiographer was in a bit of a flap and asked Bella to move around to get the baby to roll over, but with no success. We were eventually told to go for a walk up the road and see if the baby shifted. Twenty minutes later we were back – the woman was apologising and explaining that she was sure it was a girl but just wanted to be one hundred per cent certain. The baby had moved, just a little, but enough for us to get clarification – I was going to have a daughter.

Knowing the sex made it all much more real. We started calling her 'she' rather than 'it' and I think we developed an even stronger bond with the baby as we could more clearly picture our life ahead with a little girl – not that I really knew what that picture looked like. We decided not to tell anyone the gender. Although we wanted to know ourselves, we wanted it to be a surprise for our family and friends.

During the third trimester, the check-ups with the doctor and midwife became more frequent. Bella had to start taking iron tablets as she was feeling tired and weak, and her carpal tunnel syndrome continued. One of our neighbours said that she had carpal tunnel during her pregnancy and after her baby was born it was so bad she couldn't hold him; she couldn't even pick up a hairbrush. So we were a bit worried that I might literally be left 'holding the baby'.

We started attending local pre-natal classes and it was good to see a different group of people all about to do the same thing as us. I really liked the classes – I was keen to learn all about it and wasn't scared to ask questions, even if Bella was squirming in the seat next to me after I asked another embarrassing one.

At the same time as we were going to pre-natal classes, I was also going to the complementary fatherhood classes. I found these an interesting, positive 'safe space' where I could talk, listen to others and ask stupid questions without getting funny looks from the women. They were just guys sitting in a circle, so there was a lot more swearing and a lot more cut to the chase; a lot more 'What the hell is going to happen?' The guys didn't know each other and so it was a comfortable environment to share what you were thinking or to admit you were freaking out. I'd previously had the opportunity to experience men talking and listening in a circle like this when I worked for the Uncle mentorship program, but some of the other men attending this fathers' group didn't have that experience. It took a few of them a while to open up but I think they, like me, found it very genuine and useful. All the men had very different relationships and each had different concerns. I'd definitely recommend that other men talk to their friends about their experiences, but it's also interesting and rewarding to talk to men you don't know so well about what you're going through.

Bella was keen for a home birth with minimal intervention, but we couldn't afford it. I was initially scared about the prospect of doing it at home but did look into it and found that it was statistically safer – and the hospital was only five minutes away if we changed our minds. If we had still been in the UK, we could have had a home birth for free. You get looked after by community midwives who work for the National Health Service and are attached to a local maternity unit. Once you are in labour your midwife will stay with you until your baby is born, and will visit regularly for between ten and twenty-eight days after the birth.

Unfortunately, home births are not supported by the government in Australia, so it would have cost us between $2000 and $4000 for a private midwife to attend the birth, which wasn't a financial option for us. We didn't want a 'medical' birth, so we booked into the midwife-run birthing unit attached to a public hospital. It had a birthing pool, private rooms with en-suites, and fathers were encouraged to stay overnight. They provide no pain-relief options and minimal intervention, so it was perfect for us wanting the most natural birth as is possible. It wasn't our first choice but it did fit with our plan and we were comfortable with how things were going.

I was to be Bella's birthing partner but as she couldn't have a home birth she said she'd like to have a doula to support us both during labour. To me, this meant absolutely nothing, but I soon found out what a doula was. I was apprehensive about paying a doula as there would be a midwife at the birthing unit, but Bella felt she'd be much more comfortable knowing the same person was looking after her throughout the birth, as opposed to different midwives if the labour went on through several work shifts.

The doula would also be a support for me, which Bella thought was really important considering we had no family here to help out. Neil's brother told me that he had had a helper there and that it made a big difference – the doula could do practical things like getting drinks, which meant I could stay with Bella and support her. The doula would also be able to speak on our behalf about our birth plan wishes, which would be a great help when we were in the middle of a crazy new situation, especially if things didn't go to plan. The doula we chose was a midwife at the birthing unit who also attended home births privately. We had several meetings with her to finalise our birth plan and I felt confident she was going to be a great support.

Other important decisions were also being made. Our beloved kombi, our first home and adventure-mobile, was deemed unsuitable as the new carriage for our baby. We had a 'normal' car for driving to work on the Gold Coast, but it was a three-door and there was no way I could get to work in the kombi while Bella was home – the long daily commute would grow even longer. The other issue was that the back seat was not overly secure, which is important for the baby's car seat. Also, air-conditioning was not a standard feature in 1977, so the kombi had to go – but to be replaced by what?

We weren't all that keen on the 'conformador' family estate, so I started looking at dual cab utes – car-like inside but with the ute back for the runs to the tip and general stuff that I was always shifting in the van. Bella test-drove a second-hand one and she loved it. We had found our new carriage.

I started to think about parenting at this time. What would I be like as a dad? Like most people, I figured I'd be the cool dad, the kid will love me, we will have great times, be best mates and talk about everything. Being a realist I knew it wasn't going to be that easy. I started thinking about my parents and how they brought me up. I was fortunate that they stayed together and love each other to this day. I come from a traditional family unit, and my parents brought me up well. I have a university degree, no criminal record, a job, a loving wife, good health and own my own house (with the bank), which all adds up to success in the parenting stakes, as far as my parents are concerned. Well done, Mum and Dad! But what was it really like – how would I have parented a boy like me?

When I think back to my childhood, apart from when my parents dressed me and my two brothers up in kilts and shirts with frilly collars and cuffs, it was happy and busy. When I was about twelve, I felt I had outgrown my family, and was out more than I was in. Over the next few years, I believed that I was so mature and independent – only returning home every night for food, shelter and clean clothes; like most boys, I offered my parents little in return. I felt my parents were too strict – always wanting me to do my homework and study – what did they know? Life was happening outside and I didn't want to miss it.

They were right to be worried: lots was going on outside. A boy from my class was jailed for killing someone in a local park, a guy I knew died of a drug overdose, and a boy we played football with had his throat slashed walking home after a match – dead for no other reason than he had a Celtic scarf on. Looking back on those years, as a parent-to-be, I would have nailed my door shut – how can you have the courage to let go? Our baby wasn't born yet and I was already freaking out about possible risks – how can you grow to trust your children (their judgement and their luck) to come home that night? From this reflection I realised how amazing my parents had been, totally unappreciated by me as a boy of course.

Decisions about work were also upon us at this time. Bella was entitled to twelve months unpaid maternity leave and we both agreed that she should take that in full. She went on leave five weeks before she was due. I'd pencilled in two weeks off work from the due date, but told my boss it would be whenever it all kicked off – he understood.

Bella's blood pressure started to rise and in parallel her feet swelled up like balloons. Her fingers also swelled so much she couldn't wear her rings. The due date approached. The due date passed. By a few days after the due date, I felt something was going to happen every day. My mobile was face up on the table at every meeting I had. Every day I went to work I was thinking, This could be the day! Yari and Nella had just had their son, Sonny, everything had gone well for them and we were all happy to see the junior football squad growing.

It was a Saturday, four days after the due date, when Bella said she was starting to have real contractions (she had been experiencing mild 'tightenings' for a couple of weeks now). We went for a walk on the beach and Bella felt it starting to happen. Funnily enough, we met Neil walking his dog Kamu. Neil's baby was not due for over three months yet, and when we explained what was going on his eyes opened wide and he wished us luck.

The contractions continued but were bearable, so by 8 p.m. Bella decided to go to bed to try to get some rest. I had borrowed some DVDs, thinking it might be a long night and that it would be good to watch a few funny films. Bella didn't, for some reason, agree with my teenage comedy flicks and decided contractions in bed were a better option. But by eleven o'clock the contractions were strong and it was impossible to sleep. Bella spent the rest of the night walking around the house, sitting on our large blue exercise ball, leaning over the couch – anything to manage the growing pain. Each time she groaned after a contraction I would rub her back or stroke her head, then, with not much else to do, I would go back and sit down and continue watching the DVD. I felt things were going to plan – we had our bags packed, the house was ready for coming home with the baby and we were standing by to go to hospital.

At 5 a.m. we ran a bath and Bella got in, hoping to ease the pain. As she stood up to get out of the bath a bit later, her waters broke (conveniently), so I phoned the birthing centre, told them she'd been having contractions since the day before and that her waters had just broken. They told me to stay where we were and phone again when the contractions became three minutes apart. There weren't many rooms in the birthing unit and we didn't know how many others were about to 'pop', so we didn't feel comfortable until we knew we were going to get a room. The contractions did come faster within a couple of hours, so I phoned again and they told us to come in. The car was already packed with all our stuff so we drove there immediately and went into our room. We had pillows, blankets, the big exercise ball, an electric oil burner (tagged for use in a hospital), and our iPod to play music. I set it all up, closed the curtains, and dimmed the lights – just how we wanted it. Everything was going according to plan. We had phoned our doula from the house and she, conveniently, happened to be the midwife on duty at the birthing centre that morning.

We had got there at about eight, and by ten Bella was desperate to get into the birthing pool. I put my boardies on and had my camera ready. We walked across the hall to the room with the pool and stepped in. Bella's contractions were growing more intense and we were holding hands – just like I'd been told and imagined our birth would be. By about midday we were both exhausted – the contractions were full-on. The midwife asked if Bella felt as if she wanted to push (she said she had heard something in the sounds Bella was making that told her she was ready), and she did, so the pushing began. I was holding her hand, we were breathing together, and I was rubbing her back and supporting her emotionally and physically as she moved into different positions. The birthing unit had no pain-relief options so even if Bella had wanted pain relief at this point she couldn't have it unless we transferred to a larger hospital forty minutes away.

By now the nursing shifts at the birthing centre had changed, so the midwife who was on duty became our doula and a new nurse became our midwife. It was apparently all going well and the doula said she could hear in the different noises Bella was now making that I was close to being a daddy.

They kept saying to push hard – and Bella said she was – she really really was. It kept going on and on and the midwife kept asking if Bella could feel the baby moving down, but Bella couldn't. She had been in the pushing stage for over two hours when the midwife suggested that Bella might want to get out of the pool as she had been in there for five hours. She suggested a walk and a sit on the toilet as sometimes the change of position and gravity can help. As Bella got out of the pool, they checked to see if they could see the baby's head, but they couldn't. I was starting to think things were going on a bit – the midwife had said to expect the baby ages ago.

We were now leaving the pool and there was still no baby. After sitting on the toilet for ages, Bella went back to our room and onto the bed. The midwife asked if she could do an internal examination. This was not part of our birth plan but as Bella had been pushing for so long we agreed. The cervix was only eight centimetres dilated – it is supposed to be ten before pushing. Bella had been pushing all that time and it was only now we found out that she was not fully dilated. She also had swelling, which they called an anterior lip. We later found out that this means the top of the cervix swells. It happens when a woman is almost fully dilated and makes her want to push, but this only makes the swelling worse and prevents the baby moving down.

Bella was having big, frequent contractions. Her body was telling her to push but the midwife told her she must now stop pushing. She told Bella to make exaggerated 'Hoo-Hoo-Haaa' noises to try to stop the pushing, which would have been funny had we both not been so concerned. She had to stop her body pushing for over an hour – the hardest thing ever when all her body wanted to do was push. Things were now not going according to plan. I was holding Bella's hand and trying to soothe and encourage her. I didn't think it was going to be like this. This was heavy and horrific and the most intense thing I'd ever been through – I wasn't saying any of this of course. The midwife gave Bella honey for energy and then announced that she knew some reflexology that could help to dilate the cervix. Hmmm, well, it *was* natural. So the midwife began heavily massaging Bella's feet and suddenly Bella's eyes opened wide and she threw up all over me. Over my head, my hair, my wet boardies – all over me. Bella was mortified and apologetic but I assured her it was okay – and then she did it again.

Finally, Bella was fully dilated and the midwife pushed the anterior lip out of the way (and I showered the puke out of my hair) so Bella was ready to start pushing again – but nothing was happening.

We decided to get back into the pool to try there again but when Bella got up off the bed there was a rush of brown fluid – meconium – which is basically baby poo. This meant that the baby, our daughter, was now in distress and could start breathing in her own poo – which wouldn't be good. Suddenly there was a big risk and everything had changed. The birthing unit is low risk only, not equipped for medical emergencies in labour. Bella was put back onto the bed. She was crying when the doctor came in. I was all over the place. The whole pregnancy had gone so well, we felt like we had done everything right and so would be rewarded by a beautiful natural birth. I now started to realise that our plan was not on track; things were happening that were out of our control. We would have to go down a different path – one we very specifically didn't want – a hospitalised birth. Our doctor was familiar with our preference for a natural birth, but as Bella pushed as hard as she possibly could, and was encouraged to push harder still, things started to look worse. She was in agony. She admitted she couldn't do it anymore. She had been pushing for hours with no pain relief, not even gas. It was all crushing my soul – I had never imagined that it could come to this.

The doctor was feeling inside trying to find the head, but couldn't find it. This was starting to panic me and everything started to happen very quickly. Times were being talked about and procedures planned and put into place. Moving us to a larger hospital equipped to deal with emergencies was also talked about. The doctor gave us a last ten minutes to try for a natural birth, then the ambulance was called for the forty-minute drive.

Bella was put on a trolley and wheeled to the ambulance in excruciating pain and utter distress. They wouldn't let me go with her, which only distressed her further. As they drove her off, I was told to clear the room and take all of our stuff with us in case someone else was admitted for a birth. We had totally decorated the room and now I had to rip it all down and get pillows, blankets, essential oil burner – which didn't seem so essential now – and a big blue ball out of the room and into the car as quickly as I could while my wife was being whisked away in an ambulance.

I changed into dry clothes and I had a bag over each shoulder and in each hand. I had the cords for the stereo wrapped around me and throws and wraps and clothes between each finger. On the way out I was handed my camera, which I'd left in the birthing-pool room. I followed the doctor, who was helping me and was equally burdened with our paraphernalia. He dropped the big blue ball and was trying to catch it as it bounced down the corridor of the birthing unit, out of control – like I was feeling. We stuffed everything in the back of the ute and I began the drive to the hospital on my own, knowing that my wife and unborn baby were in an ambulance and in distress somewhere in front of me.

Looking back, I think it was at this point that I fell in love with my daughter and my wife on a whole new level.

Realistically, one or both of them could die due to the circumstances they were experiencing. I was behind the wheel of a ute breathing 'Hoo-Hoo-Haaa' to stop my head exploding with stress.

The on-duty midwife was in the ambulance, but afterwards I learned she didn't touch or soothe Bella once on the journey – despite the fact that Bella was writhing in constant pain. Thankfully, the ambulance crew were extremely caring and gave Bella some comfort and pain relief via an inhaler, or 'Green Whistle', which made her throw up again. Our doula was also following the ambulance, in her car, in front of me, having a lot less paraphernalia to pack and carry. That journey was the worst I've ever made. The scenario was one I had never contemplated, and I didn't know how to deal with it. When I eventually arrived at the hospital, our doula was there waiting for me and we ran through the corridors to find the maternity ward.

We had imagined a beautiful, calm, natural birth and now we were in a room with about eight people, bright lights, monitors bleeping and other things pipping and pinging. I was so not ready for this space.

Bella was crying and wondering what was happening. We had to sign forms and after they examined her we were told she would not be able to give birth naturally and they would have to do an immediate emergency caesarean to get the baby out safely. They moved her onto a trolley, which was agony for her. It was horrible; spiralling out of control, way beyond anything I'd ever considered possible – and I was feeling helpless. I was there holding Bella's hand, telling her that it was going to be okay, but inside I was seriously worried. They wheeled her down the corridor to the operating theatre and I was told I had to leave Bella and enter the operating theatre via another entrance.

I was led through a locker room where I had to put on a blue plastic hairnet and overalls and covers over my shoes. It was like getting ready to go into an episode of 'ER', except as I looked around the changing room I was startled to see centrefolds of semi-naked women – what? It seemed the most inappropriate time to see scantily clad ladies bending over motorbikes, just when I was going to see my wife cut open to save my daughter.

I came out in my new blue outfit and went into a room beside the operating theatre. A lot of people were there already dressed up for some theatre action. They had inserted a catheter into Bella and told me that she had to have a spinal block. I didn't even know what a spinal block was – I never read about any of that because it wasn't part of our birth plan. The spinal block was essentially mega pain relief and would make her numb from the shoulders down so they could operate. It's different from an epidural in that it works quickly and only lasts one to two hours.

A needle had to go right into the lower back at the base of the spine, into the space containing the spinal fluid – and it was a huge needle. Before they did it, they explained to

Bella and me that this needle goes in and leaves a small tube that they need to insert something into that they can inject the drugs through. They lock that in place and then we would be ready to go through. This is a very delicate manoeuvre at the best of times – and this wasn't the best of times. The doctor and nurses kept stressing that it was really, *really* important that Bella not move at all while this was happening. If she did move there was a risk of damaging the spinal cord. I was freaking out now. Bella was having nonstop contractions and had been for the last two hours. How could she possibly keep still? Hopefully on the surface I was looking calm and reassuring, but inside I was a mess.

They waited until the latest contraction calmed down then put Bella on her side; the huge needle went in (very carefully) and came out again leaving the tiny tube. The nurses kept firmly telling her to stay still, but I could see that the next contraction was coming – another huge one, and they were shouting now and holding her, trying to stop any movement. Bella was crying, the pain was huge, the stress was huge, and the contractions just massive and uncontrollable. There were drips of spinal fluid coming out of the tube. Everyone was super stressed and I kept saying, 'Please try and stay still.'

Bella was looking at me with tears in her eyes, completely drained and in the throes of pain, crying, 'It won't stop – it won't stop.' Again I begged her not to move. I was looking at the doctor who was to put the thing in the tube and I could see he was totally freaking out and everyone else was really on edge. Bella was desperately hanging onto the bedrail trying not to move and sobbing at the same time. After a terrifying few seconds, a woman doctor stepped in, took over and put the thing in, click, something went into the tube and as soon as she was done they all disappeared through a set of swinging double doors to the operating theatre, wheeling Bella with them. I started to follow but I was told that I couldn't go through right then and had to wait where I was, that someone would come and get me when I could go through.

Standing in that room was the most intense experience of my life. Even more intense than the journey to the hospital, just a few minutes before. I was spinning. The day had started so promisingly, but as it went on things had grown progressively worse and worse. I was numb, almost in disbelief that all of this was actually happening. We were young-ish and healthy-ish – we ate organic vegetables, visualised opening flowers and breathing the baby out, and had created a calm and peaceful environment for our baby to enter – why was this happening to us?

Now I stood alone, not knowing if Bella was paralysed after all the movement with the needle, not knowing if our baby was all right after all this time under stress and with her poo in the fluid she was breathing, or if she was even breathing at all. Just standing there on my own. Spinning. What had happened to us? Our plan was certainly not playing out the way we intended – it had completely unravelled. We were out of control and I was unsure how all this was going to end.

While I was in there, I heard Bella make a noise. I couldn't make out exactly what it was, whether it was a good noise or a bad noise. Eventually – it was probably only a couple of minutes – someone came and took me through to the operating theatre. Bella was on an operating table with a green curtain shielding everything below her chest, and her arms straight out sideways on small narrow tables. I sat right next to her head. She said she was in no pain now, and I was obviously relieved about that, but she was sobbing and so upset and scared. She was worried about how the baby was doing, couldn't believe she was having a caesarean, and was distraught that things had turned out this way. We had been up since 8 a.m. the previous day and the last twenty-four hours of labour had exhausted her. This was to be the traumatic finale.

I didn't look at what was happening on the other side of the green curtain. I didn't even think about looking. I was focused on the woman I loved and how much she had just been through and how I hadn't been with her on the ambulance ride and how she was going to miss out on the birth she had wanted. At this point, we didn't even know if the baby was still alive. The meconium had been detected some time ago now, and we both knew that was a danger.

I don't know how long it took, but it was 11 p.m. exactly when our daughter, Dylan, was born. Our original birth plan had been not to clean the vernix off the baby, not cut the cord until it stopped pulsing, and to have immediate skin-to-skin contact. But it all happened so differently. At this point, though, priorities had changed: it was about life – that was the only important thing now. They suctioned out her mouth and waved some oxygen over her mouth and nose. She made a snuffling noise and I remember the feeling of relief: she was alive – I had a daughter.

They gave her a quick rub down and wrapped her tight in a hospital blanket and passed her straight over to me. Bella couldn't feel anything below her neck, so couldn't hold her, so I held Dylan low next to Bella and we both went, 'Wow'. We told her we loved her and just stared into her eyes. It was such a relief – we breathed normally again. Bella had to get stitched up, which took another half-hour or more, and her body wobbled from side to side as they worked on her abdomen. She said it felt like someone was rummaging around inside her; as if they were washing the dishes in her stomach – very strange. It was the first time I'd held a newborn baby and it was my baby. I didn't hold her awkwardly like she was going to break as I'd feared, even though she was the most precious thing in the world to me. My arms held her naturally and safely and comfortably. I was totally in love. Eventually Bella was wheeled to the recovery room where she regained feeling in her arms, and she and baby finally had skin-to-skin contact. We put her on Bella's tummy and she climbed up towards the boob and had a good go at latching on. She sucked instinctively and we were stoked. Bella looked over at me and her whole face showed total relief: we had made it, the crazy day was behind us now and a new day and a new life lay ahead.

Our doula was sitting waiting for us to come out – it had been a very long day for her too. She told us not to worry about all the deviations from the birth plan, the most important thing was that Dylan was safe and that Bella was well. She said that during all the panic and drama the nurses had commented on how I was trying to get as much of what was left of our plan to happen – even asking if we could put some vaginal juices on the baby's head (we had been told how important this was for the immune system). Our doula now uses this story in her pre-natal classes. I hope as an example of a concerned father, not a silly man. She headed home and left us in safe hands.

Bella was taken to her room when the feeling in her legs returned, which was a massive relief to me. Once there, the nurse weighed and measured Dylan: she weighed 2.89 kilograms, which I thought was okay but apparently that's quite small and way smaller than Bella had expected. I did a few runs down to the ute and brought up the bags we needed. I had just started to set up the room when the nurse told me I had to go home. Bella didn't want me to go after what we'd just been through, but the nurse told us I had to. We begged her to let me stay but she was having none of it. After pretending to leave twice and getting caught sneaking back in, at 3.30 a.m., I had to make the long drive back home. Alone again. But at least my wife and my daughter – wow, I've got a daughter! – were both well this time.

I drove back up to the hospital first thing the next morning. Bella hadn't slept that whole night – she had lain awake with Dylan and told me that they had had the most special night gazing into each other's eyes and getting to know each other. Bella was on cloud nine and totally in awe of our new wee baby.

After speaking with a doctor, we learned that when they opened Bella up, the baby was stuck posterior (her back to Bella's back – the wrong way round) and had her chin up, so she was wedged in a position that she couldn't go back or forward from. In the wild, in the natural world, our baby would never have made it. Bella could have ruptured and both of them would have died. The doctor also said that Bella's uterus was so thin that you could see straight through it and that Bella was just about to rupture when they operated. So for all our ideology about wanting a natural birth, I felt really lucky that within forty-minutes' drive someone had the skills and equipment to save these two precious lives. Bella was so happy that both she and Dylan were alive and well, but found it hard to come to terms with how things went. She felt gutted that she hadn't been able to give birth to Dylan naturally. She was definitely traumatised by the whole ordeal and found it difficult to sleep for a long time afterwards, as the memories of the day flashed back when she closed her eyes.

The next night I went home and Neil came round for a drink – it was his birthday and so we had a good few beers and chatted long and hard in a way I don't think we had done before. I spoke to Neil that night about how I felt when my partner's and baby's lives were under threat. I realised then what I had and what I could lose; it was the first time I'd felt the intensity of love at that level. That for me was a major experience about becoming a father – feeling that love and realising who I was and the love I have for others. I didn't think it possible that I could love Bella more than I did, but after the birth I loved her ten times more. Plus I loved this other little person I'd only just met just as much. It's amazing to have people in your life who you love like that.

After two days, Bella and Dylan were transferred back to our local hospital. I drove them there very carefully, one, because of the precious cargo and two, because Bella was all stitched up. But despite being so careful it felt as if I found every bump in the road the whole way back. At the local hospital I could stay with them in their room. Dylan had a touch of jaundice and her weight had dropped due to Bella's milk not coming in for a few days, which is apparently common after emergency caesareans. I would often give Bella a rest and settle Dylan by walking around the hospital grounds with her in a sling, which was pretty cool, just the two of us, me and my daughter, her sleeping on me. It was a stressful few days as we waited for Bella's milk to come in and for Dylan to do her first proper poo. On the Thursday night I had my bag ready to go to football. I was just waiting for the nurse to come and do a test to check if Dylan's blood count had improved. She came and tested – it hadn't – Bella cried, and I texted Jim to say I wasn't going to make it to the game.

Even though the first proper poo hadn't come and we were unsure how the breastfeeding was going, we just wanted to go home. So finally, after five days, we decided to leave. The local hospital was close to our home and we wanted to be in our own space, away from bleach-filled toilets, hospital food and the sounds of women giving birth in the birthing centre. As we were getting Dylan into the car we heard a squelch – the first poo came. And what a mighty poo it was. We were ecstatic! It's funny how excited you can get about a dirty nappy.

We happily changed the nappy, drove home, and things started to became a little easier once we were back in our own environment. Things started to get hard again, though, as Bella was finding breastfeeding more and more painful. Dylan was latching on perfectly but the nurses kept saying she must not have been and that was what was causing the pain. No one seemed to be able to help and Bella was very emotional about it and was in severe pain. It was terrible to watch as she sat crying on the couch trying to breastfeed and I felt completely helpless.

She persevered for weeks and weeks, determined to make it work, and finally, through her own research, discovered that she had nipple thrush. This is a common infection that comes on after caesareans because of the antibiotics they put you on. There are no obvious signs of thrush on your nipples, however the pain can be severe, as it was in Bella's case. When feeding it felt like she was being stabbed in the back and that her breasts were full of broken glass. One tube of topical cream and she was on the mend. It's so simple when you know, and so frustrating that it took so long to get there.

Due to the thrush, we had a rough first six weeks, but despite that Bella was still unbelievably happy and loving being a mother. I was a bit all over the place in those first few weeks. Without any of the feel-good hormones that come from childbirth and breastfeeding that Bella was getting, I was tired, emotionally scarred by the traumatic events and feeling helpless about how to make Bella and Dylan feel better. There were times I remember thinking that no one ever told me that this would be so hard. But then Dylan would look at me or fall asleep in my arms or I would just watch her little legs cross and uncross while she slept and my heart would squeeze. It's hard to describe but it was a feeling of absolute devotion and awe. I had a wee baby daughter, a precious thing so needy but needed, so in love and loved.

Football was on and I caught up briefly with the boys before and after the games. It was good to be able to talk to people who had been through the same stuff. Bella and I also saw most of the team when they dropped off the food-roster meals. This was very welcome and a great way to introduce our new daughter in a less daunting way. It was especially good when Yari popped in with a beautiful thick stew and passed on the old Indian baby-calming technique: while cradling the baby, step forward one, two, three, lunge down, step back two, three, lunge down. It sounds like a school-formal dance but it worked and I in turn have passed it on to many a grateful parent.

I thought I was busy before the birth – I knew nothing! I'm not going to bullshit, having a baby is a lot more work than I imagined it would be. It is easy to see everything through rose-tinted glasses, but the reality is that it is life-changing hard work. Trying to get Dylan to stop crying was hard. Trying to get her to sleep was hard. The term 'overtired' – what a bugger that is! Where do you go from there? You assume you want your baby to get tired and go to sleep, but all of a sudden you need to know the exact moment they go from tired to overtired, because once you cross that line it becomes a whole lot harder and there's a whole world of pain ahead of you. The new mother is gifted with hormones to help her through this, but I was just really tired. I was up at night doing the settling after the feeds and the nappy changing, and then into the car and off to work, then home to support Bella who had had a full day of nursing the baby and was in need of a rest.

Before the birth, we had all these plans of how we were going to do things: breastfeeding for as long as possible, only organic food once Dylan moved to solids, cloth nappies, no dummies, no immunisations, co-sleeping, no TV, only natural cleaning products in the house and lots of quality family time. The realities hit home after a while, though, and we ended up trying a dummy after about seven weeks but only for sleep (and it worked a treat) and cloth nappies really didn't work out so we reluctantly went with disposables (they also worked a treat). Everything else, however, we have stuck to and are happy with the results.

There were so many things to learn and work out. We found that Dylan had food intolerances that were giving her a very sore tummy when she was sleeping. It took us ages to figure it out. Was it normal for a baby to make noises and bring her knees up to her chest during sleep? Some said yes, but we felt it was something that was not right. Bella cut different foods out of her own diet one by one to identify what it was that was being transferred through the breast milk and upsetting Dylan. Once we discovered it was gluten, the result was a beautiful, silent, relaxed baby all night.

A big challenge is the whole dynamic of care and the roles you each play – who does this and who does that. Obviously some things you, the father, definitely can't do and other things are obviously in your domain. I was working full-time; Bella was looking after the baby full-time – who is doing the housework? As a bloke, I don't think you really appreciate it until it happens, until you see it for yourself, how much work it is to look after a new baby. Before Dylan was born, Bella said that when she was not working, she would have time to prepare dinner and make my lunch for the next day at work. This proved not to be the case. You think there's some breastfeeding, there's plenty of sleeping, a bit of giggling and smiling, another nap, and so on. But it's not until you have to spend periods of time caring for the baby yourself that you realise how hard it is; how many things have to be thought about; how prepared you have to be just to go to the shops.

The other thing that is really tough is finances. From being fairly comfortable with two incomes we were now down to one, and all the bills were still there. We had saved some money, and Bella received some maternity-leave pay, but we soon found that we were eating into our savings and needed to work out how we could manage on one income long-term if Bella was to stay at home. There is no end to this story – we are still working it out.

Would I do it again? Straight after our birth experience I said, 'Never ever again!' But now, I'd consider it. The birth is just the beginning – all the real work starts then. It is hard and tiring but even more, it is fun and rewarding. I never knew the happiness I would get and the laughter that I would have every day with this new person in my life. Without family close by we think it is important to have a brother or sister for Dylan. We don't have a birth choice anymore – Bella has been told she will have to give birth at thirty-eight weeks by caesarean because of what happened. So the difficult, complicated, unknown birth experience has gone for us and the natural-birth option has gone too. We are still strong advocates for natural birthing, and we are glad we gave it a go. But we are just so grateful for the medical option that saved my wife and daughter's lives.

Bella was keen to do it naturally again and pushed for the medical advice to be reviewed, but when our doctor discussed it with the surgeon he was very clear that it was a major tear and that he was positive that a full-term pregnancy would be very dangerous, never mind going through labour. Knowing this, we are okay with it; again it is about what is really important and undoubtedly that is their safety.

When's the right time for another baby? I don't know. I had thought about two years apart, but some days when we were trying to get Dylan to sleep I couldn't imagine having another one to deal with too. Getting pregnant might not happen so quickly next time either; there might be more sex for longer – not such a bad thing.

Dylan has changed me as a person and my outlook on life. Rick mentioned that once he had a child he was suddenly stopping at orange traffic lights – risk-taking was no longer the natural option. I spent hours just looking at this wee thing: her eyes, her little fingers and toes, and couldn't believe she was half me, half Bella – we had made a human, a person who was going to live in this world and have her own story. I knew I needed to do everything I could to help make that the best story it could be. My focus now is her, but even in the first few weeks I realised that I could never give her what she had already given me.

I would say that there is probably another plan already in place and that we are a bit more prepared this time. I love being a dad and, when we are ready, we will take on the adventure again – all three of us. And bringing a new baby home, well, I know what it's like now. I know its full-on but I know it's worth every minute of sleep deprivation and worry because Dylan makes me so happy and I couldn't imagine my world without her.

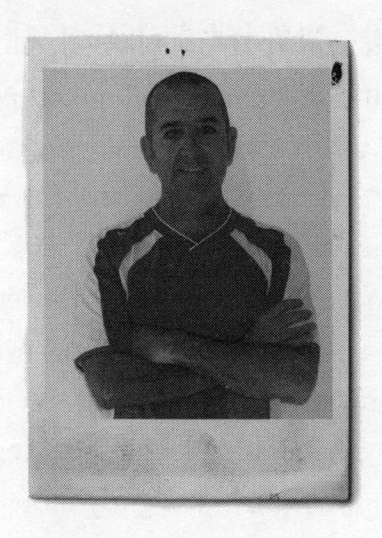

RICK'S STORY

A left-footed defender, not as quick as the younger boys but knows the game and can hit the ball sweetly. A vegetarian who's into surfing, yoga and meditation; but on the football field a tough tackler and talker. You wouldn't want to go round him and have him chasing back behind you – you know you wouldn't get far before you'd be brought down with a bang. Rick's a Bangalow Summer Sixes veteran and our inside man on the tournament, the teams and the players.

WE WERE WAITING ON A PERIOD THAT NEVER CAME. CHRISTINA had always suffered from debilitating period pain, and our whole trip to Thailand was planned around her being holed up in a hotel room somewhere for a couple of days, with a hot water bottle and bucketloads of Nurofen. We had planned to adventure over the border into Laos, to trek through a national park and live in tree-houses with a troop of gibbons for a week, but decided we couldn't risk having her period arrive while we were trekking in or out. Instead, we went for the slightly more sedate option of hiring a scooter and riding all day over the pothole-ridden roads between Pai and Cave Lodge near Mai Hong Song in northern Thailand.

Compared to me, Christina is a South-East Asia veteran and is accustomed to roughing it at times, and putting up with a bit of pain in the name of adventure. However, with the two of us on the tiny scooter with two backpacks and a guitar, eight hours on dodgy roads in the scorching heat, it was more than she could handle. When we finally made it to Cave Lodge, she only picked at our favourite meal of the local chilli washed down with a large bottle of Singha. She thought the beer tasted off, and the bumpy roads had made her a bit queasy. I thought she was just tired from the journey and would be back to her normal self in the morning after a good sleep.

The next day nothing much had changed. To Christina, the food tasted metallic, the beer tasted funny, and everything smelled bad. All this from a girl who was on the fifth trip to her beloved Thailand, and had toured India as a lone 22-year-old. She was also having crazy vivid dreams that I had run off with one of the other backpackers staying at our lodge. If you knew what to look for, it was pretty obvious what was going on, but sometimes you can't see the forest for the trees. Christina's period wasn't really late by this stage, so we put her oddness down to the heat or maybe a virus.

I grew up in Narrabeen, on Sydney's Northern Beaches. Back then, the beachfront was all fibro fisherman cottages and the area was a lot more blue-collar than it is today. Life revolved around surfing and the beach. The older guys in the water were unstable and threatening, and as a youngster if you stepped out of line you were usually brutally put back in your place.

One of four children, I was the baby by a long way, with my oldest sister being twenty-one years my senior. My brother was fifteen years older than me and left home quite early, and so I basically grew up with my youngest sister who was three years older than me, to the day. I rolled into the world and took the shine off her third birthday, and we never saw eye to eye from that day on.

My father died in a tragic accident at home a few days after my seventh birthday. Mum was left with a mortgage, and two young children. She was depressed, overwhelmed, and lonely, and she took to drinking to deal with it all. Over the next four years Mum was in and out of the hospital in an attempt to dry out and my sister and I were shuffled around to friends' and family's houses while my mum 'had a rest'.

It was at one of these clinics that she met my stepfather. They supported each other to stay on the wagon, which they did for the next twenty-five years until his death. I felt really grateful that Mum had found such a great partner, and a good man to be a father to me. Tom married my mum about the same time I found alcohol and my sister found boys. They were a really close and loving couple, and I grew up watching a perfect example of how a relationship could be.

Before I met Christina, I'd been in a marriage that lasted seven years. My ex-wife, Trudi, and I had three children together – they were all very much wanted. We had talked about having three or four, but we never exactly planned any of them, they all just appeared out of the blue when they were ready. The first time we fell pregnant we miscarried at three months – we learned that at an ultrasound. We had done the whole pre-conception thing: no alcohol, organic food, right down to choosing the best kind of soap to use. Being super healthy we felt bulletproof and the last thing we expected at the ultrasound was to find our baby had never developed a heartbeat. Having read a few books on the subject, I knew how big the baby should be at twelve weeks and when the stenographer put the cursor on each end of the foetus, it was only about half the size. I kept telling myself maybe there was a big healthy baby hiding behind the little unhealthy baby. The stenographer isn't allowed to tell you you've lost your baby, a doctor has to do it, so we were left for what seemed like hours in a cold cubicle while a doctor was found to break the news to us. We were totally shattered.

Our obstetrician advised us not to try again for six months, until Trudi was completely back into her cycle, as she had to have a curette (an operation to scrape away the womb lining) to remove the baby as it had not passed from her body the way the majority of miscarriages do. In the end we were pregnant again four weeks after that scan and Jazmine was in the back of the net before we knew it.

Jazmine was an induced birth. We'd planned to be visualising flowers, to be speaking about the petals opening; we'd selected soft music and had essential oils ready for the bath. But we were only in the hospital for twenty minutes before they induced Trudi, as they were concerned her waters had broken earlier and she was not dilating fast enough. They hooked her up to a drip and three minutes later – bam! Her eyes rolled back in her head, she pushed the button and asked for the epidural. It was a beautiful day for me, but it was also very traumatic because I had felt so useless; I could do little to help my wife who was in so much pain.

Our second child, Callum, was born fifteen months later. He was a no-drugs natural birth, born in the bath, six hours from start to finish. Our third, Olivia, arrived sixteen months after that. She was breech, which meant she was upside-down with her feet first. This was just at the time when public liability insurance was a big problem for doctors and we couldn't find anyone who would deliver a breech baby, so we had to have a caesarean section.

This was a pretty amazing birth as well. I asked the bloke in charge if I could watch. 'Only if you sit down,' he said, for fear of me fainting. I was sitting level with the curtain that had been put up between Trudi's chest and her abdomen – a bit like a tennis umpire sitting at the nets so he can see clearly to adjudicate over both sides. I could talk to Trudi on one side of the screen and watch people cutting pieces out of her on the other side. You would feel like God taking people apart and then putting them back together. By the time it was over I was so in admiration of their work that I wanted to become a surgeon.

So I'd experienced a miscarriage and three very different births: one where we were induced followed by a long recovery, one where we walked out with a baby in our arms after an hour and a half, and one where we were booked in on a certain day and time in late June. Which, as I told Olivia later, made her a Cancer, and that's why she had to be surgically removed.

After my marriage ended, I had the kids half the time, sometimes more; they were six, four and two years old. I was in a hole of pain and depression and living on eighty acres in an old farmhouse in Coorabell. I made a commitment to myself that I wouldn't let the kids down and I wouldn't go rushing off into someone else's arms and confuse them even further. Instead, I'd give myself a year to get myself together and stay away from relationships. Not that any prospective relationships were knocking my door down at this time. I was a horrible mess. It would have been easy to go to the bottom of a bottle for a few months, but I knew that alcohol manages everything badly and I needed to be at the top of my game, so I left it well alone.

Seven months into my year, I returned from a business trip and a new girl, Christina, had started work in the health food store where I picked up my lunch. It wasn't love at first sight; at that stage I was still oblivious to the opposite sex. Christina was only four months out of a long-term relationship and had moved to the north coast to live in her newly acquired caravan and to see what life brought her.

The old ducks who ran the shop had been pitching her all the prospective bachelors as each walked into the shop, and so on my return I got the same treatment. 'What about Rick, he's lovely.' They gave her the full run-down on my marriage break-up, and I think Christina commented, 'He looks a bit too old and sad for me', which at that stage I probably was.

After being in a ten-year relationship, I was just starting to remember myself again, and I picked up the bass guitar I hadn't touched since getting married. I was jamming once a week with a mate who played drums, and we had decided to go and check out a Jen Cloher gig at the local church hall one Friday night. We sat through the first support act and in the break between bands I went over to the food stall to get a snack. The girl in front of me may as well have been speaking Swahili, as the woman serving just couldn't understand her. I leaned forward and said, 'She wants a chai and a piece of lemon poppy seed cake,' in my best James Bond voice. The girl in line turned around, and it was Christina from the health food shop.

She came back and sat with me and my mate, and when we started talking she revealed she was a singer–songwriter who played guitar and was looking for a band to play with. We arranged to meet up at the local market that weekend to swap music demos so we could hear what each other's music was like. I rolled up to the markets with my demo and my three kids, and my youngest, Olivia, jumped straight up into Christina's arms without any warning.

That was it really, from then on we became good mates, hung out and played music together. We went on like that for about four months. It was at about this time that I met Christina's mate Jim. Jim was my kind of guy: he liked surfing, drinking beer and Guns N' Roses. (I could even overlook the strange co-dependent relationship he had with his dog Asha, which still continues to this day.) It was Jim who would later put together the Rusty Trombone football team and invite me to play in the Bangalow Summer Sixes competition.

I was the only one of the invitees who had played in the sixes competition before. I played in the inaugural year, four years earlier, with a team called 'Over the Hill'. Even though three of us were only thirty, the average age of the team was forty-six. We were slow and had limited skills, but the competition itself was social rather than serious. I was keen to put the boots on again when Jim asked me, and was delighted to discover that most of my team mates were as rubbish at the game as I was.

It kind of snuck up on me, but one day I realised I had started to fancy Christina. I decided to come clean about the way I felt, but she didn't react quite as I'd expected. She pretty much shot me down in flames and then rained on my parade to put the fire out.

But over the following week, the idea of us being a couple slowly grew on her. I didn't exactly fit her description of an ideal catch – a bloke eight years older than her with three kids already. She believes in manifestations and had written a list of what she wanted her next long-term partner to be. The universe will always give you what you need – but you must be very careful how you phrase things! She'd written down 'must be good father'. She meant a good father to any kids she might have in the future, not to the three others he already had from a previous relationship – but she had to admit I did tick that box.

Christina was a combined best friend and big sister to my kids and they were stoked when we told them we had become a couple and happy to see me happy again. She moved into the farmhouse with me for a couple of months and then we moved together to a larger rental where there was enough space for us and the kids when they were with us – and a big enough driveway for the caravan.

We'd only been in the new place for a month when Liv, my youngest daughter, got badly burned in an accident at my ex-wife's house. Christina and I were two thousand kilometres away sitting down to dinner at a restaurant in St Kilda, when my phone rang. I saw the number was Sophie's, a friend who lived next door to my ex. I knew straight away something had happened to one of the kids, I even knew it was Liv.

'Fitzy, Olivia's been burned,' Sophie told me over the phone. 'Burned her finger, or burned her whole hand?' I asked. 'There's been a fire and they have her in the wading pool and are running water on her. An ambulance is coming.'

Everything went slow motion on me, I tried my best to stay calm and keep my shit together. 'Is Andy there?' Andy was the fire brigade captain, he lived four houses down the road. He had heard the screaming and seen the smoke and had bolted up to the house. I had been in the local brigade with him a few years earlier. As a fireman you are taught how to assess the thickness or severity of burns, full thickness burns being the worst. You are also taught to score the area affected: an arm might be eight per cent, a leg eight per cent, the front of your torso ten per cent. Full thickness burns to twenty per cent of your body is life-threatening and a normal hospital cannot treat you; you need a specialist burns unit.

'Andy is in the wading pool with them,' Sally said.

'Give the phone to him.' Then, 'Mate, how bad is it?'

'Full thickness to twenty per cent.'

My world stopped.

It took all my strength not to lose it, the phone had been passed to someone else. 'Daddy, Daddy is that you?' It was Cal and Jaz my older two, they had been incredibly brave and were in shock but fell apart as soon as they heard my voice. The tears were streaming down my own face as I tried to tell them their sister would be okay from two thousand miles away. I knew they would airlift her to Brisbane as it was the closest burns unit. The next couple of hours were a blur of driving a rental car around Melbourne at high speed, changing flights so I could go straight to Brisbane and packing up our hotel room. In the end, we actually got to the burns unit before Olivia did as she was stabilised at the local base hospital before the flight.

When she was wheeled in, my heart broke to see my baby girl so badly damaged. At the burns unit I had to hold my naked little girl and comfort her while two burns nurses peeled the blackened skin off her for over an hour. Her ear looked like the white ash you would see in the bottom of a campfire.

Over the next ten weeks, she bravely endured several operations and loads of physio before she was released. It was great to see how many people back home offered support and help with my other two kids, and many made the two-hour trip up to the hospital to cheer up Liv. Jim rolled up with a swag of kids' DVDs for her, which helped while away the hours she spent bandaged in her bed. These days Liv is just like any other feisty seven-year-old. She's had a couple of surgeries since leaving hospital and probably has a couple more ahead as she gets older. We don't really notice her scars anymore, they're part of who she is whether she's wearing a bikini or tackling her brother in backyard footy.

Christina did so well to watch the little girl she'd grown to love go through such a lot of pain while being supportive to me and staying in close contact with my ex-wife and her extended family. There was no honeymoon period of luxuriating in love for our relationship – it was a baptism of family fire.

The other painful reality going on at the same time was that my mother was diagnosed with ovarian cancer just as Liv came out of hospital. Because I was the only one of my siblings who lived near my mum, I was her main carer, taking her to doctor's appointments, chemo and checking in on her. My mother was a very strong-willed woman and she managed to survive much longer than is usual for women with ovarian cancer. In late February, about a year after Liv had been burned, Mum took a turn for the worst and was admitted to hospital. She died on the Tuesday after Easter – being a good Catholic she didn't want to take the shine off Jesus on his special day so she hung on for one more. Shame she didn't hang on for a few more, because it was just a few days later that we found out Christina was pregnant.

Christina had only ever wanted one child, as she wanted to continue to have the time and energy to pursue her music and personal goals, and even that plan may have grown more daunting now she'd inherited three of mine for fifty per cent of the time. I didn't really want or not want another child. I didn't want Christina to miss out on what I knew was a wonderful experience, but I'd had my first three children at twenty-eight, thirty and thirty-two, and that was seven years ago now. It would be like going back and starting my apprenticeship again, wouldn't it? Maybe I wouldn't be climbing mountains in Nepal when all the kids left home after all.

We weren't really trying but we weren't taking many precautions either, so although it wasn't planned it wasn't completely unexpected when that period we were waiting for in Thailand never came. Christina was feeling sick again on the return motorbike journey from Cave Lodge. The plan from here was for me to fly on from Bangkok to London for a work convention, and she would fly down to southern Thailand and chill out on the beach somewhere. At my urging, we did a pregnancy test before we went in our separate directions. After following some crap directions down a grubby back alley, we located a chemist who sold us a pregnancy test that Eve may have used – it was that old. Nothing showed, so I was off to London.

A week later, Christina was still feeling sick. She also told me that she'd woken up the night before with an old lady standing over her. 'Was it one of the cleaning ladies in the hostel?' I asked. No, she thought it was my mother, standing over her and looking at her tummy.

We decided to try another pregnancy test, as she still hadn't had her period. I was on the end of the phone in my hotel room in Kensington Gardens as she described the two very clear blue lines that appeared. We were pregnant.

I was happy for myself but immediately concerned for Christina. She was still in Thailand and still not feeling very well. I shamefully thought, What a dirty country to have a pregnant partner in. Of course I soon realised that they have many healthy babies in Thailand and our baby was in Christina's tummy – a healthy, sterile environment – but I wanted to get her out of there as soon as possible. I should have been more concerned for our fragile little foetus previously, when it was getting shaken around for nine hours a day on a scooter (I'd even stacked it a couple of times) and while we were eating red-hot food and drowning it with Singha beer after Singha beer. Of course we'd never have done any of this had we known.

I wanted to see Christina and reassure her. She was having all sorts of concerns. Could she bond with a child? Would she love the child? Would it love her? I think it brings up a lot of relationship questions regarding your own parents and childhood when you first realise you are to become a parent yourself. When my ex-wife was pregnant with our first child, I remember going round to my mum's and apologising to her. I'd just found out I was going to be a dad, and in a short time I realised what an obnoxious, ungrateful little prick I'd been when I was young. I also began to understand the unconditional love that parents have for their children, and that they act out of love all the time. None of this had dawned on me until I was in the position to be a father. The other immediate thought I had was to do with my mortality. I started to take more care of myself, not running traffic lights or taking any type of risk. I knew that it wasn't just about me anymore. I was about to have someone who was going to depend on me and I had to make sure I would be there for them. I was looking forward to the pregnancy and birth and baby and child from the word go.

The first trimester of Christina's pregnancy was horrific. She had morning sickness like you wouldn't believe. Stupidly, it had not entered my head that this was a possibility. My ex-wife had been slightly sick one afternoon – dragging her feet on a seven-mile hike on our honeymoon – but that was all. Christina was bedridden for fourteen weeks and on a drip in hospital a couple of times. She couldn't eat, she was dehydrated, she was frightened. The baby, of course, was fine. On the bright side, Christina was the skinniest she'd ever been, and later her boobs grew bigger, so she had this amazing figure that she'd always wanted. Pity she couldn't put on her bikini and go down to the beach to enjoy it, because she was so sick.

Having been a regular heckler at our first season football games, Christina's noisy wit was missed at the early matches in season two. She did come along to one game, though, and brought my three kids with her. It was the first time the kids had watched me play, but to their disappointment, I copped a football to the face, which fractured my nose, and I spent the whole second half on the sideline with them handing me tissues to stop the bleeding.

Christina's morning sickness made it hard for me to work or do anything; I hadn't considered this at all. Sure, in eight months time she'd need my support, but right now? It wasn't even on my radar.

We tried all sorts of researched and recommended remedies – ginger, peppermint, bananas, acupressure, acupuncture, acu-everything. Then fourteen weeks to the day, she felt better and she started to enjoy being pregnant as she began to feel the baby move quite early on. With my first child, I'd read lots of books on pregnancy and parenthood, but that was nearly ten years ago. Christina, being bedridden, was reading enough for both of us and devouring book after book after book. There were a few that were lighthearted – Kaz Cooke's *Up the Duff* was funny and useful – but most books seemed very righteous and they scared the shit out of Christina.

We went to a local hall one night out in the sticks and saw a few birthing films. Everyone was lying around in bean bags and drinking chai and eating gluten-free cakes. Lots of different couples were there. Some were old, some had their kids with them to share the experience, some looked like kids themselves, and some were lesbians who must have had a sperm donor. One movie, called *Orgasmic Birth*, told the story of how some women have orgasms during birth. It showed a woman's face as she was leaning on the side of a birthing pool just after giving birth, and there was no doubt what was going on for her. This film also showed lots of stories of women having natural home births with very limited intervention.

Most helpful was a day-by-day pregnancy calendar Christina found on the internet, which showed what was happening to her and the baby every day. It compared your child to a piece of fruit each week, so one week it was a strawberry, the next week a plum, and so on.

The great thing we did do together were the Calmbirth classes. I'd been to pre-natal birth classes before, but these were completely different. We attended an introductory class and then signed up for the course, and I couldn't have enjoyed the sessions more. I learned so much – and I thought I knew a bit after having three quite different births already. Calmbirth covered in detail how the biology of the body works and how the muscles in the uterus wall work, what fear and anxiety can do to your breathing and your natural blood flow, and what your ability to carry oxygen in your blood does to your muscles. I'm a nuts and bolts type of guy who likes to know how things work, so all the background information suited me just fine.

Calmbirth gave us the confidence to strive for a relaxed birth, in which the body could work the way it should, the way it was meant to – the natural way – and not lock into the fear and the pain that's associated with childbirth. That's not to suggest there wouldn't be discomfort or that it wouldn't be hard work, just that we should not focus solely on the fear.

The Calmbirth classes completely empowered me as a man. I felt that I would be an important part of the birth; that I was needed; that I was necessary; that my contribution could help the chances of it being an enjoyable and appropriate experience; that my partner would feel safe and cared for. For my first birth I had felt as useless as tits on a bull. As a bloke I always saw myself as provider for and protector of my family. To watch the person you care about most in the world go through such a physical struggle and there's nothing you can jump in and thump, or lift up, to relieve them makes you feel quite powerless. Calmbirth suggests that one important task the non-birthing partner (me) can do, is to field and answer the logical questions that will be asked of us (using right-brain activity), while the birthing partner (definitely not me) could 'stay in the zone' she needed to be in (using left-brain activity), particularly during the final stages. The only hard part of the Calmbirth classes, held at night, was to stay awake through the guided meditations each week. I never made it once, snored a couple of times, and even had that falling dream and slammed my foot down on the floor as I fell, which scared everyone in the class and snapped them out of wherever calm place they'd been.

So we went into the third trimester calm and confident. The baby was due on New Year's Eve. Christina was big and heavy going into the hottest part of the year. She was retaining water, which I couldn't do much about, and had swollen feet, which I could, by way of foot massages. I could also get some the baby's future provisions together.

Flashback to seven years earlier and I was on a surfing trip with my mates south of Sydney. On the way home we drove past a garage sale. I was having a wander through and told the lady my wife was just pregnant. The woman took me aside and showed me her cot. She talked very highly of it and showed me how it worked and how the doors opened so you could sit next to your baby and pat them off to sleep. I was convinced. The boys were all yelling at me from the car – they weren't so keen – but I unscrewed the cot anyway and just managed to fit it in around the boys and the boards. I had that cot for all of my three kids, it was a great cot. Then I gave it away to a mate's sister who was having a baby by herself since her fella had shot through.

Flash forward to now, and when I found out Christina and I were pregnant I asked my mate to ask his sister if she still had the cot. She didn't. She'd given it to a couple who were travelling around Australia at the time. Five weeks to go and we didn't have a cot. Then my mate called and said, 'You're not going to believe this.' His sister was in Ballina that morning and had bumped into the couple with the cot, who she hadn't seen in four years. She asked about the cot and they said they were just about to move house and that it was in their garage ready to be taken away and we could have it if we wanted. So after seven years, we would be using the same cot.

At our final Calmbirth session, just after the relaxing meditation time where I'd fallen asleep again – I hoped my subconscious had heard what the teacher was saying – Christina said quietly to me, 'I'd like to have a home birth.' It was about eight weeks to go. I hadn't done a home birth before and really wanted to, and not just to get another badge on my sleeve. At the time, three out of seven midwives at our local birthing centre did home births (this was before the insurance issue with midwives doing home births).

We asked around, but no one was keen to do it. Not because we posed any type of concern, but because our baby was due on 31 December. Eventually, one midwife said she might do it, so we went to meet her at her house. She seemed to enjoy the birthing process and knew a lot about it, but she didn't take on every couple that asked her, so she was really interviewing us. She agreed to take us on, but said she'd have to ask her husband as there was every chance we'd be calling her out on New Year's Eve. I told her our baby would be a Capricorn, and that they are supposed to be diligent and on time, so we were all set for a home birth come New Year's Eve celebration.

Christina's father is an obstetrician and gynaecologist, so every time we went down to Adelaide to visit her family, he was able to give us a scan. He's done about ten thousand scans in his career, but never for his own grandchild, so he was excited. It was beautiful to see him jumping around as he saw his grandson appear on the screen. It was a different experience for me: it felt sobering to see my baby on the screen for the first time – that's when it became real for me. For our final scan her dad arranged it in 3D – it was like the 'In the Womb' TV documentary minus the Richard Attenborough voice-over. As the camera moves around you can see the eyelids, the lips, the expression on the face, everything. We had a DVD of it, which we showed to the other kids, and they roared with laughter when the baby moved his arm to scratch his arse. Christina kept one of the pictures of the baby in her womb, in her wallet.

Although her father was a specialist, we kept him out of the loop about the home birth – we didn't want to put him through the anxiety. Obviously he knows best what he's been taught – straight down the line, western medicine – and our views were sometimes quite different and 'alternative'. If we'd have allowed it, he would have had Christina taking drugs for morning sickness, for example – and we wanted a more natural pregnancy and birth.

Christina wanted to know the sex of the baby, which I had never done before. We knew we wanted to use the name Henry if it was a boy, and Ella if it was a girl, so we called it Henriella until we were sure. There was no doubt when we saw the 3D scan and Henry in all his 3D baby-manhood. A boy would even up the baby ledger for Fertile FC as well. Yari had a boy, Jim had a girl and Ross had just become the proud father of a girl, so another boy balanced both my family and my football team.

The name Henry had come about when we were walking on the beach one morning when we were first pregnant. Christina and I were with the three kids and we all began throwing around names. I've always liked old-fashioned names – names that most people wouldn't like, I suppose – you don't see too many Walters or Mervins on the streets these days. Jazmine threw out Henry and we liked that. I only knew one Henry and he was a lovely man, so the suggestion stuck.

So we had a birth plan and a name ready – all we needed was the baby. We planned a water birth and bought a blow-up backyard pool because to hire one was $400. Our pool was cheap, but big enough and strong enough so that we could lean on the sides and it wouldn't leak. We planned to put it inside our lounge room, which is on the first floor, so I had to do some research about where the beams were – half a ton of water and a pregnant lady had to be supported, literally. We had to buy a selection of hose connections to run hot water in and had a dry run the week before (but with water, so I guess it was a wet run) so we knew it took about forty minutes to fill.

We also had our birth support team selected and ready. As well as the registered midwife, we had a good friend, Penny, who also happened to be a paramedic, and another friend who does acupuncture, re-birthing, past-life regressions, and so on – a woman of some experience who has nine children of her own.

We had a meeting with our birth team and outlined how we'd like it to go and what each of our roles should be. We had a program right down to including Christina's mother and sister, who were living just around the corner. They weren't to be at the whole birth, but they would be the caterers. We'd call them and they'd bring a fresh fruit platter round. We could make the room quite dark, even during the middle of the day and we'd have essential oils burning. One thing we knew we could bank on, though, was that on match day, everything could change. For example, all the birthing mother's senses are heightened and what might have been her favourite smell when you discussed it beforehand may not be her favourite smell while a baby's head is poking out. Smell can be a very sensitive issue on the day; a birthing mother can tell if you were drinking bourbon four weeks ago. As a birthing partner, you might have to put deodorant on, then clean your teeth, and then go and take the deodorant off and clean your teeth again.

It started at about 7.30 p.m. on the eve of New Year's Eve, 30 December, when Christina's waters ruptured. She was uncomfortable. In my experience, women do look particularly uneasy just before it happens, you can watch them that day and – sorry about the analogy – but I don't know if you've ever seen a dog who's about to have puppies: they look like they're looking for something but they don't know what it is, and they can't quite see it. She had that look for about two days prior. By 10 p.m., we'd packed the kids off and rung the support team. Christina was wandering about with intent, I was moving the furniture out of the way and Penny and the midwife had all the emergency paraphernalia ready.

Part of Christina's birth plan was to make a cake. Not from a packet mix for the sake of it, but a real cake, from scratch. This is something she doesn't normally do. I understood that having another process going on at the same time as the labour would be a distraction for her. And it would also be something for us all to eat when it was over. I was quite calm. I was feeling involved and connected with Christina, and she was really in the zone. We had some props we'd collected for the pool: a plastic chair and a beach ball for her to lean on. And of course there was always me to bend into any position necessary, and not necessarily with my head above water all the time – it was a deep pool, let me tell you.

It was a balmy night and we were in and out of the pool all evening. I didn't really feel all that concerned; I feel watching any birth is a very humbling experience. I'm grateful that women do it and as a man you realise how unbelievably strong they are; they have so much strength, and it's so different from male strength. Christina was strong and calm, and just natural.

After some time, I remember looking around and thinking, Where's that light coming from? I knew we had little fairy lights and tea-lights, and candles, but this was the sun coming up; the soft sunlight on Christina in the pool looked beautiful. So New Year's Eve had started and we'd been at it twelve hours. Christina was still in the zone, occasionally bellowing deep and long. (Actually, a young bloke who lived nearby told me a few days later in the surf that he thought someone had a cow in their backyard.) I was feeling very much a part of the process: Christina was leaning on me, and I was encouraging, massaging and shaping myself to be hung onto. It's funny where a birthing woman will go to get comfortable: at one point all five of us were under the dining-room table holding hands. The pool had taken on an ecosystem of its own; after twenty-four hours there was all sorts of stuff in it, as well as Christina, me and also Penny taking a turn when my back was aching too much.

Christina was pretty adamant about having a water birth but it had now been well over twenty-four hours since her waters burst and the baby was no longer in a sterile environment and so the chance of infection was greatly increased. If we'd been in a hospital, they would have induced her already. The midwife had a word with me away from Christina: 'I can see she's not exhausted but she's not fully dilated. I think we'll have to call an ambulance if nothing has changed by 6 p.m.'

So, it came to 6 p.m. and Christina was still in the zone and working hard. It got to 7 p.m. and we had tried everything. We'd been in the pool, over the pool, under the table, over the table; we had her up and about, at one time doing something like a tribal dance, the entire support team jumping and stomping with her – it was all delirium and woman power. We finally rang for the ambulance at 8 p.m. on New Year's Eve, usually the time we'd be booking a taxi to go out.

The ambulance arrived pretty quickly – they treat it as an emergency – but Calmbirth had prepared us for this eventuality and a hospital birth experience. Christina was really worn out, and she could finally rest in the ambulance – she even fell asleep for a short while. I think she was in the transitional stage (moving from the first stage of labour to the second, pushing stage). I didn't want to be away from her. I had to chase the ambulance in a car with Penny while the midwife got to ride with Christina. We'd all been awake for about forty-eight hours; the labour had been twenty-six hours.

On arrival at the hospital we found the room Christina was in, and the nurse, who was already with her, was a bit shocked we were coming in at such a late stage. Before she could start a scene, I manoeuvred my way to the front, led the nurse away and kept any panicky talk away from Christina. We didn't think we were at any risk at all and we didn't want to be induced. Everyone and everything was moving quickly and we could see the top of the baby's head and a mop of hair. Christina's legs were put into metal banana-shaped stirrups, and she was connected to a drip. I made sure they didn't put any drugs in it to induce her even though they wanted to.

Christina was bearing down, pushing and shoving. The nurse explained they had a duty of care, and we agreed to start giving her some drugs very slowly while we waited for the doctor to arrive. Another thing we didn't want, and which we'd talked to the midwife about, was an invasive internal examination. We didn't consider it accurate, and if you think you're doing well and they say you're only dilated two centimetres, it's disappointing. A woman's cervix can go from two to ten centimetres in ten minutes or from one and a half to two centimetres in an hour.

The nurse at the hospital did an external examination and discovered Henry was on his side. She was able to manipulate him and he was out ten minutes later.

It was New Year's Eve. We were at a hospital right on the border of New South Wales and Queensland. Henry was born at forty minutes past midnight Australian Eastern Daylight Savings Time. So there were fireworks outside the window just before he was born, and then just after he was born there were fireworks again, this time from the northern side of the sky from Coolangatta, Queensland. Henry was the first baby born that year in the Tweed, Gold Coast, Byron Bay and Northern Rivers area of New South Wales, and the second in Australia.

Kevin Rudd's $5000 lump sum baby bonus had finished on 31 December, so we missed out on that by forty minutes. If we'd driven ten minutes up the road and given birth on the side of the road in Queensland we'd have received $5000 for doing so.

My first thought was, Gee, he's got big hands. He weighed just over four kilos. Christina was crying. He was so beautiful and we didn't want to break him. Even though I'd held my babies before, he felt so amazing and new and tiny and fragile. Actually, how we were holding him at first was stopping him from breathing properly and once I noticed, I pointed it out to a nurse and she grabbed him and took him off to a respirator. I think his neck was a bit constricted and he wasn't really used to breathing yet, but what felt like ten minutes was probably the best part of thirty seconds before he was back in our arms. He went a few different shades of blue – they look like little aliens, with all sorts of bluish colours and waxy mucus all over them. Some babies come out with cone heads, but because Henry had been in the birth canal for so long, his head looked more like one of those helmets that cyclists wear in the velodrome. Christina had been in labour for about thirty hours, I reckon. But when do you start the clock? When the water breaks? The first contraction? When the contractions become really concentrated?

After the weighing and testing, we probably didn't get to bed until about 2.30 a.m. – me in the world's smallest and most uncomfortable plastic hospital chair. The hospital doesn't allow partners to stay overnight but they had no chance of waking or moving me once I fell asleep.

When we awoke the media was there to see us. There were reporters from three newspapers who wanted interviews and two full TV crews. We'd slept two hours in the last fifty-eight, so weren't looking our best and our answers were a bit sluggish. Watching the news that night we appeared a bit slow and simple. We also hadn't showered for days apart from our time in the birthing pool, but we got through it and have TV footage and newspaper clippings to show Henry when he's older. We wanted to go back home as soon as possible, but we had to wait one and a half hours so they could be sure there was no haemorrhaging and Christina had to have a couple of stitches. It was the morning of New Year's Day now and all the surgical staff had long gone home. The only doctor working this shift, as part of the procedure of examination and stitching, said to Christina, 'Do you mind if I put my finger in your anus?' – now there's a question you don't hear every day!

Once discharged, Christina and I walked with Henry to the car, which I'd parked wherever I could the night before.

In the daylight I saw that that was right next to the Westpac Rescue Helicopter landing pad, and as luck would have it the helicopter came in to land just after we'd opened all the car doors and windows to let some fresh air in. It felt as if someone had an industrial-strength leaf blower aimed at our car. Christina was bent over double, our delicate little Henry in her arms, and the car was soon filled with thousands of dry leaves. The floor was inches thick with them. We were picking leaves out of the car for months afterwards and still found some more when we took the baby capsule out six months later.

On our first day at home we had visitors round pretty early, which in retrospect wasn't the best thing for us. Someone brought food over, family who were living nearby came around, all my kids were there. I think it would have been better to have had more time to ourselves to start with. But in saying that, Henry has always been very social and has loved having people around since then. I took him down to the beach that first day. Christina waded away from me and dived into the ocean and I gave him a quick christening on his first day on the planet by blowing air in his face to make him close his eyes and mouth and then pushing him under a small wave.

Since then, the best thing about having a baby is … just watching him. Watching him do anything; build with blocks, knock blocks over, blink his eyes, move his arm, even just breathing in and out. I watch him play and I'm so focused that I forget where I finish and he starts – that's the best thing. They are just perfection; their eyes and nose and ears; everything is so new.

I've been lucky, but sleep deprivation is a big challenge. When your partner is breastfeeding there's not a lot you can do to help at night, but your sleep is disturbed anyway. I used to lie awake listening to Henry breathe. Every single silence is a worry, then you hear them roll over and smack their lips and you relax. We had him sleeping in the same room as us so he didn't need collecting or taking back to another room. If there had been any illnesses or abnormalities early on, that would have been a real challenge: colic, jaundice, etc. I'd had that before with one of my other children. With Henry, Christina had real trouble breastfeeding. She had mastitis, which is blocked milk ducts that get infected, and got very sick as the infection went through her body. The early days had been fine; we initially had some success and took for granted that it was going to work. But, as can often happen, the baby stopped latching on properly and that caused problems. But to her credit, again, Christina stuck at it. I know I wouldn't have.

I have always seen myself with four kids; maybe because I'm one of four myself, and Henry is, like me, the youngest by a few years. But Christina loves being a mother so much that I might end up with five or six. Now that I'm back in the baby stage again, and enjoying it so much, I'd love to have another one.

Unconditional love is a powerful thing. If you never have a child, you don't know what you're missing out on. You'd throw yourself in front of a bus for them the moment you lay eyes on them. Being a dad is life's greatest gift for a man, especially once you've seen how hard it is for some people to even get pregnant. It's always an adventure. It's definitely something I was ready for, but it's still full of surprises. Every time I start to think I'm on top of this dad stuff, someone moves the goalposts and I realise that even after four kids, I'm still a rookie. I know a lot of blokes who are unsure whether they'll make a good family man or not until the baby comes along. Don't doubt yourself: enjoy the experience and be involved – see yourself as an important part of the pregnancy, childbirth and child-rearing process. Your kids need their dad, and dads need their kids.

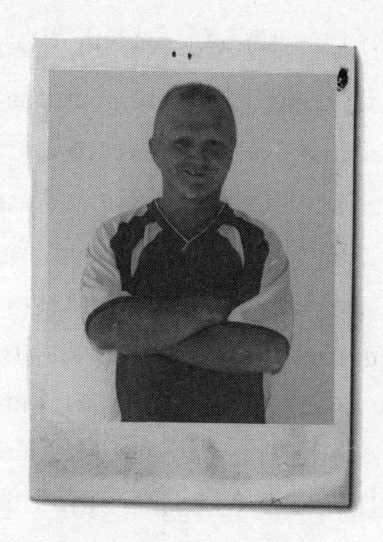

NEIL'S STORY

A short man with a big presence on the field. A bit too round and a bit too old, but Neil has obviously played some football in his day. Nicknamed 'Rock Solid', because his defence is more tenacious steel than technical skill. The amount of shouting he does at his team mates makes up for the yards he can't do himself, but he's always first to shake the hands of the opponents and usually first at the bar afterwards. He's the oldest member of the team by far, yet carries knocks well, and never seems to get badly injured. Neil doesn't warm-up (he doesn't see the point of running if you're not being chased or chasing something), preferring to save his energy for the game. He doesn't warm-down afterwards either, preferring to soak in an Epsom bath at home with a glass of red wine.

I GREW UP IN LONDON, AND WAS SEVENTEEN WHEN PUNK WAS AT its peak. I had safety pins in my school uniform, an inclination towards rebellion, and a season ticket to Tottenham Hotspurs FC. Twenty-five years later and living in Australia, I still felt I was living life like an outlaw, but crossing the road before the light goes green and not shaving before work was my feeble rebellion. I was in my late forties, still able to take advantage of opportunities (mainly because I didn't have kids) and still loved watching football. I watched English Premier League and European Champions League games live on TV in the middle of the night, and when I couldn't watch them I'd tape them and watch them as soon as I could, before finding out the result.

One 'important' European Cup final between Manchester United and Bayern Munich was shown at 2 a.m. in Australia, but on this particular night I had to take an overnight train to Sydney from Byron Bay (where I lived), for an audition for a TV commercial. I had, rather smartly I thought, arranged for a friend of a friend in Sydney to tape the game so I could pick up the tape when I arrived early in the morning, find a friend's place with a VCR and watch the game before my audition in the afternoon. I had a shower at the Salvos at Central Station, picked up the tape and started phoning around actor mates in Sydney to find a venue to watch the game. Actors aren't the most reliable of people, nor the wealthiest, and I could not find anyone who had a VCR that worked. I was walking up George Street, wondering where

NEIL'S STORY

I might find a videotape machine, when a flashing neon sign lured me in.

I walked up the stairs and smiled at the man behind the counter with my videotape in hand. 'Can I watch this on one of your machines?' I asked the porn-shop attendant. He looked at me quizzically and outlined the complete range of sexual alternatives he had on offer that would, no doubt, make my recording inadequate. I explained my situation, and fifteen dollars later I was sitting on a plastic chair in a tiny cubicle with only a box of tissues for company, watching Manchester United score twice in the last few minutes to win the game. I'm sure my shouts from the cubicle surprised the late-morning customers as they perused the shelves in the shop behind me: 'Come on boys, one more, you're nearly there!'

I had a very happy childhood, with great parents who stayed together regardless, and one brother two years younger than me, who I've always been the best of mates with. I was named Neil Young – a famous name – and there have been times in my life when I've been reminded of it. Neil Young was the Manchester City FC football player who scored the winning goal in the 1969 FA Cup final in England. It was 1–1 against Leicester City when Mike Summerbee crossed the ball from the right-wing and Neil Young met the ball in his stride, lent back and blasted it from fifteen yards into the back of the net – that's the stuff that dreams are made of.

I was nine years old and sitting on the floor of my grandad's house in the East End of London watching the game on a black-and-white TV with the rest of my family. There's also a Canadian folk/rock singer called Neil Young, but as far as I know he never played football.

I disappeared from England when I was twenty-four, just about the time my mates started disappearing with nice girls to 'settle down' with. I now know I left England because I didn't want to just meet a local girl, move somewhere a little bit nicer, do a little bit better than my parents and then have children. I think it happened to most of my mates – they became their parents, really quickly. I wasn't smart enough to know that I'd be happier living my own life first, but I was lucky enough to have the opportunity to travel with the work I was doing, and smart enough to realise that I wouldn't be very good at the 'settling down' thing right away. I was working for an international management consultancy firm and I asked for a move to work overseas, imagining getting to know Spanish or French girls. A vacancy came up in Sweden, so it was Scandinavian girls I would try to get to know.

I played football for an English pub side in Stockholm, the Tudor Arms, and at the pub met my first wife, Pirjo, who was Finnish. We were happily married for thirteen years but never had kids. She didn't want to. Her mother was an alcoholic and Pirjo had brought up her younger brothers and sisters, so I think she felt she'd already been a mother of sorts. She once said that having children was what couples did when they were bored with each other, and I understood what she meant.

I'm glad I didn't have children early in my adult life as it gave me the opportunity to fully pursue my own direction, desires and dreams. I thought I knew what I wanted at twenty, but I was young and wrong; then I really knew what I wanted at thirty and I was closer; but now, nearly fifty, I'm really, really sure I know what I want – and I can only hope I'm right at last. I've discussed it with friends, and I think a lot of men only have children because their partner wants to – we have to agree with the woman's body clock. If she wants to have children in the next couple of years we will, if she doesn't want to have children, we won't – it would be wrong to deny her that choice, wouldn't it?

When you first fall in lust with someone at the bar or in the bedroom or wherever, you don't ask that question – you don't ask if they'd like to have children at thirty-two, or thirty-eight, or never. And then by the time you've been together for a while, you've fallen in love with them, and it's too late to have that conversation.

When the cold and dark of Sweden wore us down, we were able to move to Australia with my work. We arrived in Sydney and loved it, but eventually bought a house in Byron Bay – this was before the real estate prices around there went ridiculous. I starting working part-time and pursued an earlier dream to study acting. We got a puppy, but still we drifted apart. Four years later, at the age of forty, I was a once-divorced, childless, unemployed actor, living in Byron Bay with my dog, Kamu.

Like lots of actors I knew, I was usually earning money doing something else. I was working from home doing graphics and still 'consulting' for the international firm and occasionally going back to Scandinavia to run workshops and training programs for local staff. At one, in Norway, I met Mette.

Mette was a tall, beautiful Norwegian. Three things I wasn't. She had a cute nose, great legs and laughed at my jokes. She wore jeans and trainers to work, while the other girls wore skirts and heels. She was great fun, could drink heaps and loved to stay up late talking. As soon as we met, we had great fun, drank heaps and stayed up late talking. Although there were thirteen years and a different culture between us, we liked the same music, had a similar punk philosophy and shared the same sense of humour.

Over the next few years, whenever I returned to Norway to run similar sessions, which was at least once a year, I would meet up with Mette, and we became closer and closer.

My relationship with Mette was initially long-distance, then she came to visit me, then she came to stay with me while she finished her studies, then we realised we wanted different things and she left. The lyrics of every love song I heard were suddenly relevant, and sunsets were torturously beautiful and endlessly lonely. By the age of forty-five I was

NEIL'S STORY

a twice-heartbroken, unemployed actor with no children, living near Byron Bay with my dog, Kamu.

Then, a year later, Mette wanted to meet to see if we still had feelings for each other and maybe even a future together. I wasn't sure, but I was keen to meet. We met awkwardly at the airport, and came back to my new home.

I was living in Mullumbimby, fifteen minutes from what was becoming the party town of Byron Bay. I didn't need that anymore, I wanted something different. Mullumbimby was a country town filled with country folk, but also accommodating a mix of other blow-ins including eccentrics, ex-hippies, and ex-city dwellers. My name, Neil Young, wasn't so unusual here if you considered I had massages from Keith Moon. Like Nimbin, Mullumbimby, undeservedly, was probably best-known nationally for the marijuana that was historically grown around the many banana plantations (there is a hairdresser in the main street called Mullum Heads). Rumour has it that a few years ago, when some Mullum folk heard on the local radio that sniffer dogs were in Byron Bay assisting arrests for marijuana, they immediately organised to spray the entire main street with bong water, so by the time the sniffer dogs arrived in Mullumbimby they didn't know where to sniff, until they found a pump-action water pistol in a rubbish bin.

I think Mette was impressed with where I was now, geographically and emotionally. We settled into comfortable chairs on the deck for a chat and, at that moment, I knew what I would say and do in the next few minutes was going to have a big outcome on the rest of my life.

She said something like: 'I'd like to be with you ... if I come here and we make a go of it, then I'll be giving up everything ... we'll have to get married for me to stay ... and ... I want to have children one day.' This was said over the duration of a whole evening, of course, although I'm sure she'd been practising on the plane.

I was involved in the conversation as well. But while talking I was thinking, Could this be the right relationship, or the right time? Or both? Now that there was the prospect of having children one day I got a little excited – although I must say, when there had been no chance, it hadn't bothered me.

So Mette moved to Australia and moved in with me. We took all the furniture out of the house, cleaned the place, and then moved all the furniture back in together so that it became more our space than my space. She did well to find a job in Byron Bay in a real-estate office, and within five months we got married in a small personal ceremony with close friends from Sydney on Wategos Beach, as her visa and our destiny dictated.

I started playing football with the Rusty Trombones when we'd been married for about eighteen months. It was also around this time that I first started hearing, then hearing more and more, 'Neil, I really think I'd like to have a baby.' Mette was thirty-five, I was forty-eight.

Gradually, my smiles became nods, and eventually nods became smiles and nods at the same time. We decided to try properly after Christmas. We were going to have a big New Year's Eve with Ross and Bella, then I'd stop drinking and smoking, so my mature, but keen, sperm would have the best chance on their long swim. I don't think I had doubts about them making it, but I wanted them to be as fit as they could be. Mette started taking fish oil and came off the pill – this was a big thing for sure.

What's the best way to get pregnant? Well, here's a good tip for beginners: have lots of sex. We had *lots* of sex. Every morning and every night for a week, and before, during and a week after the most fertile times. Happy days. This was very different from our usual dance of one of us initiating sex every so often. Mette was now ready all the time, she'd give me the look and off we'd go again. At one point she said I was like a wild animal in bed – but unfortunately I knew she meant the muddle I made twisting in the sheets sleeping during the night. We laughed during sex – for all the right reasons too. We tried it this way and that, had pillows under the bum, hers and mine, and held her ankles up in the air and shook them. By the end of a monthly session I was totally exhausted and, I must admit, pretty happy for it to come to an end and to get some more sleep.

This was after our first season of football but before our second. Jim and Sarah were pregnant and we knew others in the team were trying or 'not not trying'. It took us three months to get pregnant – sometimes I wish it had taken longer, but other times I don't know if I could have lasted many more months. Inexplicably, one morning Mette got up and said something felt different inside her. It was the morning after. She had certainly always wished it and this time definitely felt it. She took a pregnancy test far too early, but then took another about a week later to confirm what she already knew.

The morning I found out for sure, I already knew it was going to be a stranger than normal day when a bird flew into our bedroom window. There was a dull thud and I got out of bed, shook off the blanket of last night's memories and went to see what the noise was. The bird lay there stunned and wide-eyed. I picked her up and moved her to somewhere safe where the dog wouldn't bother her and later she flew off for the rest of her life. It was also to be the first day of the rest of my life.

Mette was in the bathroom doing another pregnancy test and I was sitting on the sofa. She came out and told me she was pregnant. I remember saying, 'Wow', and seeing her face change from the girl I loved, into the woman I loved, who was now growing someone inside her. Without a doubt, my life also changed forever from that moment. I visited a strange place where you feel love, trepidation, love, fear, love and more. I quickly ran a short film in my head – it was a montage of birth, baby, child, school bus, sports day, and more. We cuddled and giggled and made tentative plans about something we knew nothing about. We saw a doctor for the first time at four weeks; he wasn't as excited as we were. He told us it was best not to tell anyone for ten to twelve weeks as that was when the greatest risk of miscarriage would have passed. So we told no one. Except Mette's family in Norway, of course; and close friends overseas and interstate; also Ross and Bella – they'd told us they were pregnant before their twelve-week deadline, only a few months earlier; and my brother, who now lived in America; and my mum, who now lived in Australia, close to us. Then we were out at lunch a few weeks later with some old friends (who we also told), when one of our best friends from Sydney phoned to say he and his girlfriend were pregnant, '... it's only eight weeks, but anyway'. So I put my hand over the phone, told Mette, and asked if she minded if I told them.

I'm not sure if I actually did this, but I thought of writing a list of everyone we'd told so that if something went wrong I could call them all and tell them before they asked us how it was going. It's so stupid not to tell friends and family. If you do have a miscarriage surely that's when you'll need the support of friends and family most – rather than pretending nothing's happened. It seems like a hangover from the Victorian times when you didn't speak about anything that happened down your trousers or up your skirt. However, it was nice to tell special people in a special way and say, 'You know, we had to tell *you*, but please don't tell anyone else. There's only sixty-four people who know, I'll add you to my list.'

I didn't tell anyone else in the football team, but I remember watching a European Champions League football final (Barcelona won) at my place late one night with Jim, Yari, Ross and Nick. Jim already had a baby and Yari and Ross were out of the closet with their pregnancies and enjoying a new male conversation about how wonderful it was and how fortunate and amazing it was that their babies were both due at the same time. Nick and I were sitting listening while watching the football, and I knew Mette was pregnant too, but it was too early to tell them – they weren't on the list. I got up and went into the bathroom where Mette was getting ready for bed and said, 'Metz, can I tell them?' She said no. So I didn't. But I so wanted to. I don't know what Nick was thinking.

I finally told Jim when I was helping him move house a month or so later. As we were carrying a cabinet out to the removal truck, I casually dropped my news. Jim already knew, I'd been too coy around the campfire on the surf trip and Mette had asked too many questions of Sarah at the pre-season training picnic. Jim said she had looked so comfortable holding his blond, blue-eyed daughter, Bijou, that Mette could have been mistaken for her mother.

Soon we settled into the routine of the first trimester. And our routine was morning sickness. And what an erroneous name that is. It doesn't just happen in the morning, it happens all day! Mette had an intimate relationship with the two largest white things in our house – she either had her head in the fridge or the toilet. I also thought her moods varied between slightly and extremely unpredictable and irrational. A friend had a fortieth birthday party around this time and the invite said to come as something 'freaky'. There were ghouls and monsters and capes and platform shoes and I went, on my own, as a pregnant woman in her first trimester – the freakiest thing I've ever experienced by a long way. The costume was a good excuse to get into a frock of course, and with a small cushion up the front, a wig, some lippy, and a big L-plate on my stomach I thought I looked the part. To others though, I looked like a sad, desperate transvestite out on his/her first date, and my outfit was met with weird curiosity and sideway glances, I didn't meet many new people that night – maybe it was me who was unpredictable and irrational.

Having to eat certain things at certain times is very difficult, but during Mette's pregnancy junk food was okay anytime. It's not easy hearing your lover barfing over the toilet several times a day and although not much good food seemed to stay down, apparently the baby takes what goodness it wants and will not go hungry. Our baby wouldn't go hungry for sure, especially if we kept going to Hungry Jacks as much as we did – and the nearest one was over half an hour away. It could have been worse, though. Yari told me someone he knew had a craving for dirt wiped off a car. And Nick said he knew someone that used to suck the plastic of the shower curtain. Well, maybe fast-food hamburgers were okay.

During these early stages of pregnancy we were also renovating our house, doing our best to change it from a groovy bachelor pad to a groovy pad with a nursery. We needed to add a home office (we were both working from home doing graphics but currently sharing the same desk) and another bedroom and bathroom, so there wasn't just one of everything. Luckily, we had space underneath the house to spread out the way we wanted to. But this was all done while Mette was feeling sick, and while the house was being re-stumped. I was able to stand in our kitchen upstairs, shift my weight and move the whole house, which didn't impress Mette at all. She had to move to my mum's for a few days while walls were sanded and concrete was polished. Occasionally, Mette would come downstairs where we were working and say, for example, 'Why did we get these windows? They'll be hard to clean.' 'Well, darling, some of the reason is that you weren't available when we were choosing them and specifically told me to go away and sort it out myself.'

We were reading books about pregnancy. Every Sunday morning we would lie in bed and I'd read about the particular week we were up to in our pregnancy. The baby is the size of a shoehorn, is starting to grow nails and can close its eyelids – that sort of thing. Mette would listen and I'd read, it was really nice. We had two books and we'd read the particular week's chapter from both books – one was *Up the Duff* by Kaz Cooke and the other was *Your*

NEIL'S STORY

Pregnancy Week by Week by Professor Lesley Regan; one serious and factual and one more lighthearted and easy to understand and relate to.

Our thoughts on the type of birth we wanted were based on our different cultural backgrounds. The decision was, of course, mainly Mette's and I'd support whatever she wanted to do. Coming from Norway, Mette was used to birth being a hospital procedure and really didn't mind the idea of a caesarean. Yet now she was living in one of Australia's centres of 'alternative' thinking. We talked to lots of alternative people, were offered lots of alternative advice and read lots of alternative books about alternative options – mostly very natural. Our birth plan was 'have a healthy baby' – however best that was to happen. We went to see a midwife at the local hospital and as Mette was not a high risk we were told we could have our baby naturally at the birthing centre. Mette was comfortable with that, and I thought it was a great idea.

We had 'shared care' – alternative appointments with a midwife then a doctor every two weeks. I thought that was great too. We felt well supported and cared for. We also attended Calmbirth classes where we did breathing exercises together to stay calm, confident and not let fear enter. Male support at birth was a big part of Calmbirth. By identifying a space where the mother-to-be felt safe, you could use shared imagery to calm each other if things got a bit scary. Mette chose her safe space: that moment when you first go underwater when scuba diving, when it all goes quiet and the tranquillity of the underwater world opens up in the sunlight from above.

We also did pre-natal classes. These were run by nice midwives who told us useful things we didn't know about: breastfeeding, colours of poo (with pictures handed round) and folding cloth nappies. For one exercise, while the mums-to-be were doing something vital, the boys were sent off and had to write on a big sheet of paper all the 'things that will change when you have a baby'. Well, 'fucking everything' is the right answer, but I'm not sure we knew that then. The classes were a good process to get us focused, and gave us some essential knowledge. To start us thinking, we were given a questionnaire with questions like, 'Will you let your baby/child see you naked?' – things we'd never considered. The classes were also a chance to meet other pregnant couples in the area who were going through the same experience. Along with the football team, it widened the circle of people we had more in common with than friends we'd known for years who weren't pregnant.

Mette was in much better health in the second trimester and we spent a lot of time together. We watched a lot of DVDs, our last chance maybe. We watched a whole series of 'Grey's Anatomy' – twenty-three episodes, three to four hours a day, on a weekly hire – all about hospitals! We stopped doing Lotto when we found out we were pregnant. After reading books about the odds of having a birth defect or a problem at birth, however slight, I wasn't able to wish to be in the one in a million who wins the lotto. I just didn't want to be the one in 1500 who has a baby with a birth defect, particularly as I was an older father, which increased the chances of an abnormality.

Choosing a name was a big thing for us, particularly Mette. She spent an incredible amount of time looking out for names in books, magazines and on the internet. We'd watch the rolling credits at the end of TV programs and DVDs more intently than the show itself, scanning for a good first name amongst the cast and crew. She mostly had girls' names in mind because she wanted a girl. I went to sleep every night for weeks hearing lists of girls' names, and got quite good at going, 'Mmm, mmm, nhhh, mmm, nhhh' in my half-sleep. One book had the romantic suggestion that 'she' could be named after where she was conceived – India, Paris, or Lucia. We weren't sure how happy our daughter Bondi Couch would be about that if we'd conceived on a party weekend in Sydney.

I'd always wanted to give my child the middle name Danger, especially if it was a boy. Like a James Bond character: 'Danger is my middle name ... no, really, it is.' What a pick-up line. What a gift to my son. However, there is a tradition in our family that the firstborn has the middle name of the father (our firstborns were all male), so my father was Geoffrey Joseph Young, after his father, Joseph Picton Young, and my name is Neil Geoffrey Young. Additionally, my father was big on acronyms, and wanted to call my brother Kay Ann (if he had been a girl) Young, so that his initials would spell Kay, the first name. Following this logic, I suggested the name Andy – it had it all, Andy Neil Danger Young – brilliant, I thought. I may not have come up with as many suggestions for names as Mette but at least mine were thoroughly thought through. Suffice to say, Andy didn't go down well, and Mette craftily knocked it out of the running by naming a possum that visited our deck Andy, so that that name was now used – I couldn't name my son after a possum.

Mette wanted to know the gender of the baby, so at our second scan, at eighteen weeks, we found out it was a girl. I have really only known boys in my life. I grew up with one brother, and I'd worked for many years at Uncle – a mentoring and activities program for boys without active fathers – and had been mentoring a boy since he was nine, sharing time with him on weekends. I hadn't known a little girl since I was a little boy, and although I'd always got on well with girls, the female psyche was something of a mystery that I'd been spending most of my adult life trying to understand. To use a football analogy, I felt as if I would be playing away from home, and wasn't sure whether I'd brought the right boots.

Looking back at my time with Uncle is interesting. Was I drawn to that organisation in my late thirties because I realised I probably wouldn't have children of my own? The boy I mentored is now a successful young man in his twenties, but I didn't really fill a father role. As he said, I was 'More of a mate, but a mate who happens to be thirty years older than me.' I knew nothing about being the responsible guardian of a girl, though. I really hoped I'd got the right boots.

Having a dog was good practice for having a child, I think. It's like the exercise where teenage girls who want to have a baby are given a raw egg to look after for a weekend. They have to make sure it doesn't roll off the washbasin while having a shower, or drop it while carrying shopping, and see if they can bring the unbroken raw egg (the same one) back to school on the Monday. I think not breaking a dog is good practice for not breaking a baby. Kamu was a golden retriever–lab cross and we were together for thirteen years – my longest relationship. He taught me some great qualities, like the bumper sticker says: 'I'm just trying to be the man my dog thinks I am.' I thought that's what fatherhood would be like. Feeding and caring for another life takes time, it's an investment, but the rewards make it well worth it.

Anyway, I was really looking forward to getting to know the gentleness of a little girl. And now we only had to choose a girl's name, that halved the possibilities. We decided to bestow on her some English and Norwegian heritage, and used our grandmothers' names Grace (English) and Helene (Norwegian) as middle names – if only I had a grandmother called Danger. The first name was still to come from the 'Top 20' list and more names were added as more got crossed off over the following weeks.

We discussed vaccinations around this time and heard both sides of the argument. Where we live, in Northern New South Wales, the immunisation rate is much lower than elsewhere in Australia. We are lucky enough to have a choice, but given that choice, it makes it really difficult. We concluded that if we chose not to immunise we were making a choice primarily for our baby, and if we chose to immunise we were making a choice primarily for society and our community. I'm happy we took the decision for the community. The way I see it, many diseases don't exist today because of high immunisation rates, and if we all make personal decisions then fewer people vaccinate and some diseases will reappear. We decided we would take what we considered to be the path of least resistance and would do all vaccinations as recommended by our doctor.

With three weeks to go to the birth, at our regular midwife appointment, we were told that the baby was breech. This was the same situation Jim and Sarah had with Bijou six months earlier – the bum near the exit and the head furthest away, with the feet next to the forehead. If she stayed in that position for another three weeks, it would either be a difficult natural birth or a caesarean. We were told that with an external cephalic version (ECV) – an injection to relax the uterus – and a medical massage, it was possible to turn the baby around, and that there was someone local qualified to do this. We both quickly agreed that it didn't seem very natural to push our baby around from a position she was quite comfortable in, and further, there was a risk of the cord getting caught around her neck. Our doctor said, quite frankly, that it depended how much Mette wanted to feel contractions and have a natural birth – back to the birth plan: 'healthy baby', safest option and path of least resistance. So we decided to wait and see if she would turn by herself and if not we would have a caesarean birth.

This meant our Calmbirthing would go out the window, but hopefully not the baby with the bathwater. We were encouraged to use some of the techniques we had learned from Calmbirthing including the safe space underwater imagery of scuba diving. An elective caesarean meant that instead of going to the local birthing centre for our final couple of check-ups, we went to the much larger hospital with its corridors, queues, stainless-steel doors and sick people, to meet anaesthetists. There were tears; it was a difficult transition for us to make at first. I felt that Mette and the baby's safety was most important and we should take the advice of the experts. I was also a bit relieved to know it wouldn't be so much of an unknown and unpredictable experience for Mette.

Elective caesareans were performed on Wednesdays, so we could choose the fourth or the eleventh of February. We chose the latter as it was only three days before our due date, and as this was Mette's first birth it was 'unlikely' that she would go into labour early. Interestingly, if we'd chosen the other date, our baby would have been born on Ross' birthday – and Ross' daughter was born only an hour before my birthday. Also, our daughter would have come into the world the same day my father died seven years earlier.

We had finished playing football in December. Most of the team members had gone through their birth experiences and I'd heard all their stories in detail when we met delivering meals to them in their first week. The closer we came to the date, the more comfortable we both felt. I really enjoyed the last few weeks. We knew exactly what to expect. At home we were ready, but it was weird having baby clothes in the house and a room ready for someone who didn't exist yet. Like when someone dies and their clothes are still there but they are never coming back to put them on. So there are these little jackets and socks, all washed and folded and ready and no one yet owns them.

Now that we had a planned date for the following Wednesday – 'No sorry, I can't meet you for lunch today, I'm having a baby' – we could relax and have a great last weekend together as just a couple. We had breakfast out on Saturday morning and enjoyed it so much we did it again on Sunday morning. We watched a DVD on Monday night with a pizza, then had an early night on Tuesday – the last time we'd sleep together as just the two of us – knowing that in the morning we would be driving to the hospital to have a baby.

We got up, got ourselves ready and packed a bag with clothes for someone we hadn't met yet. We had a standard, new-parent station wagon (with room for a pram), and had been driving around for a few weeks with an empty car seat in the back. But this was a new feeling, like going to pick someone up, someone who was going to stay for a while. We drove calmly up the coast. It was a beautiful day, but there had been bad bushfires in Victoria. We had to be there at 8.30 a.m. but weren't going to have the procedure until 2.30 p.m.; there were many tests and pre-op procedures to be carried out beforehand. We were shown to our room, which had only one bed in it, so we didn't have to share with anyone – not sure if we were lucky or not, but we were definitely grateful. We spent the day talking happily, discussing names and taking photos of ourselves together, with the camera at arm's length – that was going to be harder to do when there were three of us.

The worst part of the whole operation (says I, the person not undergoing surgery) happened in our room just before we went into the operating theatre. Mette had to have a catheter inserted so she could pee. I realised quickly that it was horrible to watch someone you love in pain, and I hoped the rest of the day wouldn't be as painful. Apart from that though, the build-up was calm. Mette was calm. Calm people came in to check things and give her things and take things away. Mette completely understood what was going on and I felt we were in the right place with the right people.

As our time approached, we were told twenty minutes. Deep breaths, Mette. Deep breaths, Neil. Scuba diving – sunlight flickering through the water from above. Love you.

Soon, the sides of the bed came up with a clank and we were off, out the door and down the corridor to the operating theatre with people on every corner of the bed, including me, and the one midwife who was on shift all day with us. It was good to have someone constantly there with us who we could build a trusting relationship with.

As we went through the banging double doors, I was led away to put on a blue plastic suit with elastic around the wrists and ankles and a blue shower cap. I also had strange blue plastic shoe protectors over my thongs. I put these on in a locker room, I suppose where the doctors get changed. Then I thought of what Ross told me, I looked up and saw pictures of half-naked woman, like pin-ups from a mechanic's shop in the seventies. Ross was right, how very strange.

I was led out, still a bit stunned, in my blue plastic suit and met Mette sitting sideways on a trolley about to have the spinal block inserted. Apart from us, there were about six people in the little anteroom before the double doors of the operating theatre. Most were behind Mette preparing scary looking tubes and needles. A lady next to me said she could take our camera; she said she'd seen this dozens of times and knew the best places to take snaps of us. I'm sure she had a job to do and wasn't there just to take photos, but there were so many people I wasn't sure who was doing what, even though they did all introduce themselves.

One of them inserted the needle for the spinal block and told Mette not to move. I was supporting her at the front, she was leaning on me. Another lady next to me said, 'Neil Young, that's a good name, do you get teased a bit about the singer called Neil Young?' I tried as best I could to strike up a conversation with her, but didn't really have my heart in it to explain about the footballer Neil Young. Mette asked me to concentrate on supporting her and of course I did, but it was strangely social. I guess it's a normal work day for them.

We heard a baby scream from the operating theatre. Scream in a good way, like 'Hello world'. It must be the one before us – gosh they seem to do this really close together. With the spinal block inserted, Mette was laid on her side, made as comfortable as possible and wheeled off through the double doors into the theatre. I was told to wait a few moments before I could go through. They all left and it went quiet. I was suddenly on my own without Mette or my new friends. I wondered if any man had ever turned and run at that moment. Soon enough, someone came to get me and I was taken into the operating theatre.

It was bright and sounded like a party in full swing: there was soft-rock radio blaring out and the room was filled with even more people than before, all milling about industriously, chatting and preparing unidentifiable things. I felt like I'd arrived late to the party. Mette was the centre of attention and was lying with a green curtain across her chest. I went and stood where I was told, next to her head. People had started work on the other side of the curtain, but she couldn't feel anything from the chest down. I didn't dare look. Mette said she was feeling like someone was pulling hard inside of her. I did what I could to keep her calm. She was calm. I'm not sure I was. We were told by the lady holding the camera (who I then saw did have another job alongside the anaesthetist) that it was almost over. We'd probably been in there twenty minutes.

Suddenly the movement, chatter and clashing of surgical instruments increased and then, just as suddenly, a small squealing baby was carried head-high from Mette's tummy to a little table where she was wiped and wrapped in a blanket. I was taken over to cut the umbilical cord, which I did – it's tougher than you think – in sheer disbelief as I looked at our baby daughter. I started crying uncontrollably, and I heard a particular song on the radio that I swore to remember for the rest of my life and play to my daughter one day – I forgot it five minutes later.

Our new daughter was brought over to us. She still had a bit of stuff on her face and was a bit squidged, but she hadn't been pushed through a birth canal, so she looked perfect. She was placed on Mette's chest and I got in close for our first photo together. We spent the next few moments just staring at her, talking to her, smiling at each other and crying. Forget religion, this was a miracle. We were in such a place of love.

Meanwhile, Mette was tidied up behind the curtain. We weren't asked and didn't want the placenta, thanks. Some friends of ours who had a baby at a birthing centre had dropped off their placenta to us after their birth as we had the nearest freezer. We had that placenta in our freezer for far too long and eventually returned it to them at a barbeque – making sure to remember which bag the sausages were in. Mette was stitched up; this took some time but we were with our new baby so nothing else really mattered right then.

After about another twenty minutes we were ready to go, and I tried to thank as many people as I could before we were taken into another room and our baby was unwrapped and placed naked on Mette's chest for skin-to-skin contact. As soon as she landed on Mette's stomach she started to move her head around to look for a nipple, which she found after a few beautiful minutes of silent encouragement from us – incredible to watch. 'Incredible', 'astonishing' and 'amazing' are words I hadn't used for some time, but I had the feeling I would be using them all quite often from then on. It was so incredible just looking at her and thinking that Mette grew her in her tummy. She grew her bones, her eyes, her nails, her beautiful little face, everything. Love. Love. Love. Incredible.

We were taken back to our room and settled down for the first time, just the three of us. Mette was immediately absolutely smitten. I don't think I've ever seen her so happy, she was oozing love. The party girl of the past had gone and in her place was a beautiful responsible mother. The baby slept for a bit but Mette wasn't sleeping. We discussed names and, now that we'd met her, we chose Zoe from the names we had left to choose from. We just couldn't stop looking at her: perfect little fingers, perfect little toes. Even, after a few days, a perfect little birthmark on her thigh, just like her mum.

It is important that a baby does their first poo to pass any meconium ingested from inside the womb. We knew this would be black and tar-like and probably not smell very good. During the first afternoon, a nurse came in to check on us and unfortunately my eggy breakfast got the better of me and I did a little bottom-burp. Mette and the nurse were elated. 'I think she's done a poo,' they gushed.

'No, I don't think she has.' I blushed as I tried to wave away the evidence.

Too soon, day became night and I had to leave because hospital policy decreed that fathers weren't allowed to stay overnight. I drove back home in a daze. I sent an SMS to the football team and other friends and relatives: 'All good. All very, very good.' I spoke to my mum, who was so excited for us. I was feeling great. I was feeling I'd changed. I'd changed profoundly emotionally. I needed to change physically too – I got a tattoo the next day.

Back home, sitting alone in a house filled with baby stuff was a bit odd. Ross came round and we had a few drinks, as we had when he returned from the hospital when his daughter was born. We talked deeply but not very articulately about the experience. I was feeling high. I slept well, even though it felt strange being in a bed on my own for the first time in ages. The next morning, I picked up some things for Mette and drove back to the hospital.

Their first night together had gone well, although I don't think either of them had slept. As the reality sank in, and a few people came to visit, our attention moved away from the birth as an event, and towards the everyday management of this new little person. There were heel prick tests, hearing tests and reflex tests. It seemed the biggest chance of Zoe having some weakness or allergy or rash at this time was if it were hereditary. Nurses and doctors, when presented with a sick baby, will always ask, 'Is there any history of this in your family?' So my advice to any man who hasn't chosen the mother of his future offspring yet is to find out, on an early date, whether your prospective partner has a family history of skin disorders, irregular breathing patterns or rare diseases of the internal organs.

We learned how to change Zoe, how to bathe her, and Mette continued to learn the best way to breastfeed her. All the time talking quietly to her and touching her gently like only a mother can. Incredible.

That night I had to go home again. Mette and Zoe were going to have to stay in hospital for another three to four days to make sure everything was okay, as is normal procedure after surgery of this type. The next day they were to be moved to a shared room so we decided to leave the hospital and spend the last day and night in our local hospital instead. So our first parental duties in the real world were to put a new nappy on Zoe, dress her, put her in the carry capsule, take her out to the car, put her in the car seat and drive her to our local hospital – lots of firsts there for Zoe. And us.

I remember in my thirties, time used to go really quickly. Now, with a baby, it seems to go really slowly, which is a good thing. Our time in the local hospital was very much like that. As I could stay in the same room, we slept in the same bed, all three of us. The midwives helped us with bathing and feeding and time passed slowly. The first day and night at home were strange, of course. We hadn't done this before, but Zoe didn't know that, so we bluffed our way through and I don't think she noticed. We were awake most of the first night trying to settle her and then when she was quiet for more than a minute or so we woke her up to make sure she was breathing. We thought she was scratching her face in her sleep and wanted to put mittens on her hands. We didn't have any, but we did have lots of socks, so Zoe went to sleep in the middle of the first night waving little socks on her little hands.

My overriding memory of that time at home is love, love, love. When Jim came around for his turn at the meal roster (great homemade chicken burgers from Sarah), he said the scene was very surreal. Mette and I were both dressed in white, the sun was streaming in and we were both beaming with love and pride. Jim said Zoe looked like a little angel in Mette's arms.

Even in the middle of the night, pacing up and down the living room with a non-sleeping baby was usually a loving experience. The words to 'Rock a Bye Baby' are so wrong. I sang it so much I was able to workshop new lyrics, changing them so the baby didn't come crashing down to earth in the cradle. In her inside world, Zoe was used to sleeping while Mum was walking about and then waking at night while Mum was sleeping. Now we had to teach her that in the outside world it's the other way round. We had to teach her to sleep.

Every father I've spoken to says, 'I knew it would be harder than I thought, but I didn't think it would be this hard!' I thought it'd be about an eleven, but in our case, we found it to be about a seven – which was a nice surprise. We used our version of 'sleep training' and it mostly worked out well for us, with little crying and discomfort. It certainly could have been much more difficult. I suppose each baby is different, and if we have another it might be so, but for the moment Zoe has lulled us into a sense of (maybe false) capability and is therefore more likely to get a little brother or sister at some stage. Mette is so in love with her new daughter that she doesn't know how she could ever love another child as much. As a mother, it was immediate and unconditional love, while I must admit that for me, it was more about falling in love with Zoe as I got to know her.

Now, months later, we feel we are getting on top of it. We have learned how to treat each other in this new dynamic and so we're thinking of changing that dynamic and doing it again. Everything's going along so nicely, and now we're considering the possibility of a second child. A friend who has two young children told me that when one child was taken out for the day by a grandmother, all of a sudden the house seemed quiet as it was filled with *only* the sound and energy of one child. We're still grappling with the enormity of one child, and he considered that a holiday! I think some women miss having a baby once their child is a toddler and no longer as reliant on them. The most common reason I hear for having a second child is so that the first child has a sibling, but I'm not sure that's a good enough reason – it makes the second baby sound like an accessory. We'd love another, but I'm grappling with my own issues regarding my age: I'm almost fifty now, would a second child be healthy? I feel so lucky and I don't know if I want to complicate that by having another roll of the dice – you just don't know.

At its most profound level, having a baby has given me a reason for living. It's like having a project that is really important and will never be complete, but wanting to see it out as far as I can. I don't drink and smoke like I used to, I'm much healthier now. I have a good reason to try to live as long as I can. I have reason to believe in the future; to save the world; to save the environment. I have reason to believe and have faith in the human race – now I feel I'm really a part of it.

Your child becomes your life. And your life becomes good, pure, fresh and untainted. It doesn't matter what the weather's like, who's won 'MasterChef' or even whether your football team won or lost – your life is good because you can do what you love all the time: watch your baby develop and change. Watching her sleep is remarkable. Making her smile is wonderful. It's getting better and better, and from talking to the other boys in the team, I've heard it continues to do so.

Of course there are challenges. The lack of sleep is not comfortable, but it is manageable. I had more trouble with no longer being able to do everything on my terms. 'My time' disappeared. No reading another chapter, or painting, or yoga or any of the small jobs around the house I kept promising myself I'd do, because now I definitely don't have the time or energy for them. Also, it was a blow losing the undivided love and attention of my partner that I was accustomed to. She used to think I was the most fantastic person in the world – now I'm the second-most fantastic person in the world, which is still pretty good, but the competition's living in the same house. I struggled with a massive feeling of being unappreciated. I had to be a provider first, then a father when I could be present. Mette was focused on the baby all the time and I had to earn the money to allow that to happen. If I, as a father, had an opinion about the way something might be done, I didn't feel it was always valued; it was as if Mette were the only expert. That said, I know Mette had feelings of being unappreciated too – we had to find time and a new way to communicate with each other, to compliment each other as often as possible to keep morale up when we're both feeling tired and run down.

Family is important. I think lots of families today are spread around the country and around the world and so friends take on some of the role of family support. Other mums at mothers' groups become aunts and friends of dads' become uncles. My mum, Sally, moved to Australia seven years ago when my father died, and we are lucky to have her living close by (the next nearest relative to either of us is in Europe or America). I can see how it would be hard with no family network to help look after a newborn while the mum is having a shower or a wee. Sharing Zoe with my mother feels like I'm giving her something back as thanks for having me. She absolutely loves her role as grandmother, and we can see how important it is for Zoe. I only wish my father was still alive, and Mette's parents were closer so they could spend more time with Zoe, although they have made the effort to visit us and were overjoyed to meet her. Mette speaks only Norwegian to Zoe and hopefully she will pick the language up and be able to understand her maternal family. Zoe has Norwegian baby books, so I hope we can learn Norwegian together – currently our levels of understanding are about the same.

The one piece of advice I would give any man contemplating becoming a father is 'dare to be great'. I heard a tennis commentator say that about Lleyton Hewitt, after he'd played only a mediocre backhand. To do better he just needed to 'dare to be great'. I'm not sure about the sports psychology side of it, but I think this term can apply to fatherhood. You're just an ordinary bloke but you can become a great bloke by how you bring up your children. Dare to be great, step outside your comfort zone and have a red-hot go. Having a baby to rear is the best reason I can think of to try to be the best person you can be all of the time.

ANTONIO'S STORY

There was one other member of our football team during season two whose story we haven't told in these pages. We didn't stick around to share beers after the game as we had during our first season together. This meant we didn't have the chance to share our stories with him or really get to know him, meet his partner or understand their situation. They were also pregnant before the season began, and due around the same time as Ross' and Yari's partners were; but tragically their baby, Antonio, did not survive after birth.

We knew very little about exactly what happened and out of respect for the families involved we have not used the parents' names. However we did want to mention it here as it did happen and it does demonstrate the wide variety of outcomes that are possible when giving birth. According to the Bonnie Babes Foundation – a non-profit, volunteer-based charity that supports families dealing with pregnancy and birth loss – in Australia, one in four pregnancies ends in miscarriage, stillbirth and neonatal loss. (Although only one in 140 babies are stillborn and about the same neonatal, just after birth, usually when premature.) None of us knew this during our pregnancies. The difference between the worst thing you can imagine and the best thing you can imagine are closer than you think.

When we heard about Antonio we were all shocked and felt helpless and didn't know how to contribute in any meaningful way – something that is so intense is difficult to comprehend. It was devastating to hear about, let alone imagine actually happening. Jim took the lead as captain and sent out an email to the whole football team letting everyone know the shattering news and asking for a donation towards some flowers to send to the family. He also suggested that, because Ross and Bella were still in the hospital with their newborn, we shouldn't worry them with it then. Unfortunately he didn't take Ross off the group email list before he sent it, so we did all find out at the same time.

When Antonio's father came to play football with us a couple of weeks later it was an awkward time for us all. We didn't know how to convey our feelings or say anything helpful or constructive. Some of the team had just had babies and had been through a similar experience but with a polar opposite – joyful rather than devastating – outcome. I for one was still expecting a baby and could only wonder and worry further about any risks involved. Everyone offered him their condolences as best they could. Just before the game we stood around in a circle with our hands or our hips. He brought out his mobile phone and showed us a picture of his baby son. We could only bite our lips and shake our heads in sadness.

'Don't worry about your baby crying at night, boys,' he said. 'Remember, a baby crying is a beautiful sound.'

Season Three

The Trombones FC

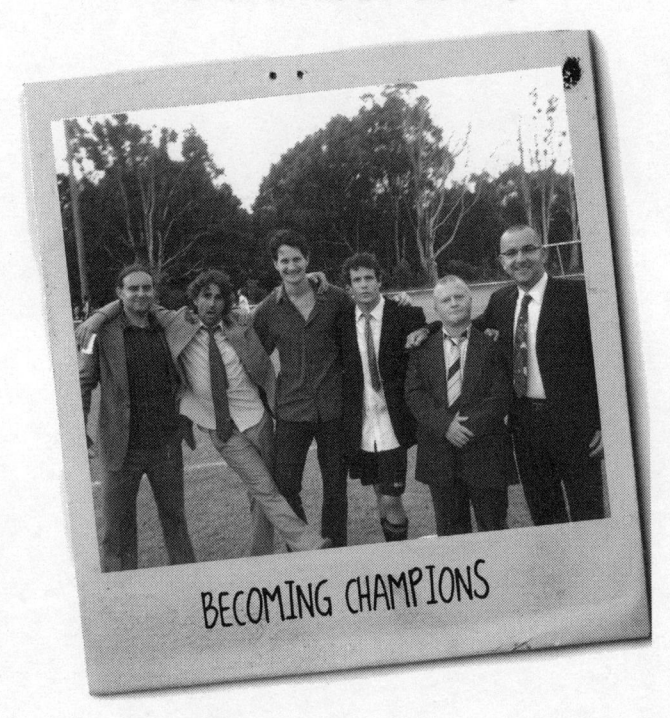

BECOMING CHAMPIONS

THE TROMBONES FC

JIM WANTED TO PUT THE TEAM TOGETHER FOR ANOTHER SEASON, and we were all keen. Looking back, we could see how we had hardly known each other during our first season, compared with how well we knew each other now. Our first season had been a laugh and we had become a football team together, our second season had been good fun and we had become fathers together, and now we were about to embark on a third season and didn't really know what it held, or what we expected – on the field or off.

Apart from the obvious highlights during the second season – the births of our children – we had played some very attractive football and hoped to continue doing so. We were fitter and we were having more fun because we were better players. From Jim's drills we knew that passing the way we were facing, making triangles, and passing then moving, was the way to play. We knew the other members of the team better and were willing to work harder for them. We had fewer late nights (but less sleep due to babies) and fewer drinks, because we went home straight after the games (and needed to be straight as soon as we got home). We wore proper shin-pads and we didn't tackle as recklessly (apart from Rick) – we had become more responsible.

In seasons past, it was as much about the social time afterwards as it was about the football before. But by our third season, we had grown as footballers and also grown emotionally as men, and valued ourselves more. We were a little older and wiser through the massive change that had happened to each of us. We still had lots in common while chatting in the car on the way to games, but it was now less about bravado and more about babies.

If the name Fertile FC was appropriate for the second season, then for the third season we should have called ourselves Completely Knackered Sleep-Deprived L-plated Fathers FC. We didn't feel comfortable calling ourselves Fertile FC, not when we weren't with pregnant partners – it seemed a bit ... boastful? After not too much deliberation, we decided to call ourselves the Trombones FC, a reference back to our inaugural season together as the Rusty Trombones FC but without any of the unnecessary sexual innuendo – although explaining the name of our team could still be awkward. Somewhere in the world Ezza and Pirate Steve were still giggling.

Five babies had been born within seven months of each other around our second season, when we were Fertile FC.

SEASON THREE

At our first game of season three together as the Trombones FC, Jim and Sarah had a fifteen-month-old girl, Bijou; Yari and Nella had a twelve-month-old boy, Sonny; Ross and Bella had a twelve-month-old girl, Dylan; Rick and Christina had a nine-month-old boy, Henry; and Mette and I had an eight-month-old girl, Zoe.

As well as these new supporters, once again we were going to need some new players, so we could share our new parental responsibilities on a Thursday night when needed. Chad was going to play another season. Chad, 'the Energiser Bunny', had so much energy that sometimes he used to drive early to games with his bike on the back of his car, cycle home again and then run the ten kilometres back to the game. He'd play the match (running around more than any of us), and then drive home afterwards. I know I was getting exhausted doing ten minutes of stretching as a warm-up.

We briefly recruited Tony, the boss of a mate of Jim's. Tony, who had three grown-up children, was now in another relationship and father to a two-year-old and a two-week-old – so he met all the requirements to join our team. We were to learn later that he was actually the man who had fallen asleep in Jim's pre-natal classes. He came to our first training session and showed some rusty skills, but after less than half an hour, limped off holding the back of his ankle – we found out the following day that he had torn his Achilles tendon. He didn't play again – ever! The poor bugger was on crutches for several months. He told us he had to help look after his two-week-old baby by scooting himself around the house with his one good leg, in his office chair.

So we still needed more players and eventually recruited Peter, a naturopath – a draft not from the pub, a rival team or a friend-of-a-friend but from pre-natal classes. He had an eighteen-month-old son and a new baby on the way. Then Jim met Ben, an old friend of Yari's, at a garage sale – Jim was always very good at making friends quickly. Ben had a two-year-old and his wife was pregnant. He would be our specialised goalkeeper, so we wouldn't have to take it in turns to put on the soggy goalie gloves filled with someone else's sweat. In true Trombones style, Ben had never played football before, but proved to be an outstanding addition to our team.

For our third season together we decided we needed a new strip. Rick organised that and we had 'Trombones' emblazoned on the front of our new red shirts. For the same price, we could also have our own name and number on the back. Hmm, what an opportunity! Should we have Jim, Yari, Ross, Rick, Neil, Nick, and so on, across our backs, or use our surnames like real professional footballers? Rick decided he wanted to be named Ricaldo, because it sounded as if he were a better footballer. Quickly, as the emails spread, we decided we'd all rather be better footballers ... and why not Brazilian footballers? So, for our first game in season three as the Trombones FC, all nine of us trotted onto the pitch in our smartly matching shirts – Jimerio, Yario, Rossaldinho, Ricaldo, Neiliniho and Nico along with Pedro, Chadalinho and our new goalkeeper, Benjami.

As we became fitter and better we didn't seem to get as sore after the games anymore, but as Rick pointed out, perhaps it was because we were smarter and had worked out how to run less. Some of us had been playing indoor soccer between the six-a-side seasons, which we thought would give us a fitness and skill advantage, but playing with a football-sized tennis ball on a netted indoor cricket pitch was like being inside a pinball machine with nine other competitive men and, apart from the joy of football, the main things we came away with were unsightly weeping grazes on our knees and thighs from the artificial playing surface.

Rick and I were forming a formidable team in defence, with more than sixty years of football experience between, unfortunately, only the two of us. Nick was growing more confident with every game and Jim was running midfield. Yari was improving in huge leaps and bounds and Ross went from scoring one goal in season one, to being in the top ten on the competition's 'sharp-shooters' list for season three (he even got a hat-trick against the Chefs).

Maybe because of the Brazilian names; maybe because we were better footballers; maybe even because Jim's uncle joined us for our first game (he was in town for Jim's wedding and had previously played football professionally);

anyway, for whatever reason, we won a few more games than we lost in season three – a new experience for us. It was a nice feeling, this playing well, scoring goals and winning.

It was about this time that we realised it didn't really matter how many games we won during the season. Each team was always pitted against similar opposition for the final series and we really only had to win the last two games for a chance to compete in the final. We also realised that we hadn't won a game in the final series of either of the last two seasons. At the end of this season we ended up in the third division and so were due to play a quarter-final, then maybe a semi-final and then possibly a final against other teams that had finished in the same part of the table and were therefore of about the same standard as the Mighty Trombones.

For our quarter-final we played against Where's Fifth on the pitch nearest the canteen with everyone watching. As we sat on the sidelines doing up our boots, putting strapping tape on and filling in the team sheet, Jim reminded us that this was where the Chefs had sat, as supporters, watching us, in the first quarter-final we played in season one. It seemed such a long time ago. We had grown so much since then, as a team and as individuals off the pitch.

Our opponents on the other team had not grown, in fact they were short one player, which made it a pretty even game of their five against our six – and we also had three fresh substitutes who could run on as fit replacements. We out-played them, Ross scored two, and Chad scored the goal of the season by lobbing over the keeper's head from way out. We won the game 3–0.

For our next game, the semi-final, the Trombettes were home tending to our offspring. Tony came to watch us; he was still on crutches from his pre-season injury. Rick joined him on the sidelines, now also on crutches. He had injured his hip two games before on the same pitch. We had all seen Rick, in a tackle, fly into the air, become horizontal about a metre off the ground, and then go straight down – hard! He was down for a while – we thought he was winded – a sub came on and we played the last two minutes of the half. At half-time he was moving a bit and was keen to start the second half so he didn't stiffen up. He only lasted about five minutes before he came back off. This was not good. He watched the rest of the match from the sideline.

After the game, Rick was strangely un-thirsty and had become a paler shade than was healthy. He insisted he was fine – he had to fly to Adelaide in the morning to meet Christina and Henry. After a bit of resistance we helped him over to his car. It was either his hip or leg, we weren't sure, but it was bad and he needed to see a doctor. He opened the back of his van, took out his mobile phone and his medical insurance card and dialled Christina's number. To say he was woozy would be an understatement, this was further confirmed when he put his medical insurance card to his ear while waiting for an answer.

'I'm driving you,' said Ross. 'No arguments!'

Talk about a team effort – getting Rick into Ross' car was a mission. Rick wanted to do it on his own, and he explained through gritted teeth that it was really sore and so he was sorry, but if anyone was near him he might lash out. We all stood back and watched as he manoeuvred himself in stages into the car – it was a painful sight indeed. At the hospital, getting Rick out of the car was twice as hard as getting him in. Ross managed to swivel him onto a wheelchair then into the hospital reception. An orderly now had the unenviable job of getting him from the wheelchair to a hospital bed. Even with the 'Green Whistle' painkiller, the orderly got the same stark warning of violence – 'Sorry mate, I know it's your job, but I might take a swing at you.'

The doctors examined him, took X-rays and put him on morphine. Rick relaxed and became quite chatty. He asked the doctor, 'I've got a morning flight to Adelaide – what's the chance of me getting the plane?' 'What month?' was the coy response. Ross replied to all the texts from the team asking how Rick was doing, then headed home as Rick couldn't move and would have to stay in hospital overnight.

Ross stayed in touch with him and finally got an SMS the next afternoon: 'Looking good for a 6 p.m. check out if that suits.' When Ross picked Rick up about twenty-four hours after the tackle, Rick was still in his Trombones football strip, had heavy medication in his hands and crutches under his arms. Once out of range of the hospital Rick revealed that he had checked himself out against the doctor's advice. Ross took him home and helped him up the stairs. Rick said he was fine, that he was going to take a shower then have a lie down, so Ross left. The next morning Ross texted Rick to see if he was okay and needed anything to be brought round and got the reply: 'Sorry mate, in Sydney, couldn't tell you or you would have been in trouble too, flying to Adelaide in an hour.'

So now we were to play in the semi-final against the Miserable Gits without Rick. They were an older side with old tricks and a few new dogs sprinkled amongst them. We had been thinking about the game all week – especially when we paced up and down trying to get our babies to sleep. And even more so after getting a 'rev-up' call from one of the other boys. The idea was that each of us had one other player that we were responsible for psyching up for the big match. By giving regular rev-up calls it would get us in the right mental frame of mind for winning the semi-final of the competition. Now, this sort of motivational management – especially screamed – is highly effective if the player is on his way to the game in question. It is less beneficial if that player is in the supermarket shopping for yoghurt earlier in the day.

Also during this week of psychological preparation (but naturally, no physical training), Rick collected motivational speeches from across the ages and oceans and sent us all hilarious emails with strange montages of mixed metaphors.

Subsequently, we rose to the occasion. We played well and it was definitely worth the 'two four-legged men' coming to watch us. We beat the Miserable Gits 4–1, although, like our previous opponents, they were also one player down for the entire game.

Anyway, to our great joy – and surprise – we had made it to the Third Division Soccer Final of the Bangalow Summer Sixes. Immediately after the game we smiled happily at each other and together went with cold beers to watch the other semi-final to see who our opponents in the final to come would be.

After watching Borange win their game comfortably, and look very impressive in a tidy orange kit (and, it has to be said, very impressive out of the orange kit as well – six-packs were seen, and variously envied or dismissed), we decided that we should dress up for the final. We would all wear suits and ties before the game, with our football kits on underneath, and step out of our suits simultaneously and run straight onto the pitch. How better to reveal our intentions, and our Brazilian brilliance? Like a secret weapon, just before we played in the final. Some of this was because we thought it might intimidate a bunch of young opponents who admired neatness; some of this was because we realised we might never play together in a final again and that we might as well make the most of it, and the rest of it was because it was just silly and would make us laugh.

The final was to be played the next week, followed, as

every year, by an awards ceremony at the local pub. We arranged for a trombone-playing friend of Rick's to come along and play on the sidelines during our final.

Obviously, we had explained the importance of the evening to our loved ones, and to their credit they understood and gave us all permission to go and play. To their even greater credit, our loved ones also understood that we would probably want to 'play' afterwards, too, and have a few drinks together after the game. Therefore we were all given the whole night off from our usual fathering duties, so that we could go back to Nick and Sally's house to celebrate if we won, or commiserate if we lost. (Sally, the only partner without a kid, went to stay with Jim's partner, Sarah.) This would be a rare occasion when we weren't required home until morning – when we smelled better.

On the night of the finals, we turned up individually (pretty revved-up from our rev-up calls) and mingled amongst the throng of other players in other finals and other supporters and friends. We found each other easily. We were the only people wearing suits and ties. It was 7 p.m. and still about twenty-four degrees on that mid-week December evening in rural Australia. The green playing fields of Bangalow looked magnificent from the high vantage point of entry near the canteen. Eight floodlit, half-size football pitches had games going on. There were about a hundred people playing and at least the same amount of players, friends, families and dogs watching. The whistles from the refs and the cheers for a goal could be heard distinctly through the summer night air.

We'd like to think we looked intimidating in a fun way, rather than stupid in a stupid way, as we tore off our ties and stepped out of our suit pants. We'd also like to think we stood a chance in the game ahead, but deep down we had our doubts. The other team, Borange, looked impressive with a ball, and were equally unimpressed with our childish behaviour as they continued to warm up. They looked faster, fitter, younger and stronger, and were probably better footballers. If we were going to be Third Division Champions, we'd have to win by wanting it more and working harder together as a team than our opposition.

Before kick-off, looking around at our team, we could see the determination and the nerves on each other's faces. We were a little intimidated, as all the talk had been about how these blokes were better than us. We were fed a rumour that they thought we were shit, except for one bloke (Jim) – well, we thought that too. We also thought that they would think Rick was our professional manager as he shouted instructions at us from the sidelines in his suit.

It was a hard-fought game. They passed the ball around well and we were chasing the ball around a lot. The first half was a tense affair, with no one giving anything away. The game began to get a bit niggly, probably because they were wondering what they had to do to score. Then it came, just before half-time and against the run of play – a Borange player was tackled in the middle of the park, Jim received the ball and found Ross on the left wing, Ross controlled it nicely with his left foot and took a shot with his right. Goal! Quickly, bring on half-time.

The half-time whistle blew. The score was 1–0.

The half-time team talk focused on how we couldn't believe we were winning 1–0. Jim said we needed to focus on defence for the second half. We were all pretty knackered already, but keen as. So, as we went out for the second half, the plan was to defend. The plan fell by the wayside after less than five minutes. Borange scored. A mishandle by Ben gifted them a soft goal and all the hard work was undone. But our heads didn't drop. We continued to work hard for each other and ran ourselves ragged protecting our goal and trying to attack their goal.

The full-time whistle blew: 1–1.

As we discovered in our first quarter-final in season one, if a game is drawn after normal time, the rules of Summer Sixes dictated that both teams play on until a goal is scored (the 'golden goal'), but with each team removing one player immediately, and then removing one more player every two minutes.

The other games had finished and more players and spectators, including the Chefs and the Zeppelins, wandered over to see how our game would end. The few Trombettes who were able to be present were quite quiet, probably because they were so excited and nervous. We were now completely knackered but still keen. We understood we just needed to score before they scored in order to win. Jim chose the team to go on while the others watched from the sidelines with the growing crowd. We kicked off and Jimerio passed to Rossaldinho. Rossaldinho tried to take a player on but lost the ball. A Borange defender passed across the pitch from the right-wing to the left-wing but he didn't put enough power on the pass. Jimerio sprinted over and just intercepted the ball before a Borange player got to it. Jimerio took a touch towards the line, then a slightly heavier touch down the line. A defender came towards him. He feigned a cross with his right foot. The defender jumped in the air to block the cross and Jimerio pushed the ball forward, under the defender, just enough to line up a shot on goal with his left foot with his next step. Bang! Jimerio connected sweetly with the ball. It went through the keeper's legs and crashed into the back of the … GOOOOOOOOOOOOOOOOAL!

We went a bit crazy after that and started running around like chooks with our heads cut off. Jim ran from the goal back into our own half and jumped into my arms. The rest of the team were close behind and smothered us. Soon we were swamped by other players and friends from the sidelines, including Pirate Steve from season one. Jim was lofted into the air as our goal-scoring hero, our team captain and the man who had taken us on this journey together. We were all in a place of absolute exhilaration, exhaustion and relief. A rare place to be indeed, but a place each of us could now relate to, having known it in entirely different circumstances only recently.

We did it.

After extra time, Trombones FC won 2–1 and became Division Three Champions.

We really did it.

We had grown from novices in season one to champions in season three – and not only as a football team, but as individual men too. When we first met, we were ordinary men with the usual self-centred and self-preservation instincts, but now we'd learned to think of others more highly than ourselves. Before we had babies, we had little real familiarity with responsibility. Now we'd learned that responsibility is not something to hide from but to embrace. We were striving to be a team of champions and now we were a champion team.

After the cheering, the grins, the hugs and the compliments all subsided, we got our stuff together, put our suits back on, and headed up to the pub to be presented with our trophy. Jim was hobbling a bit by now, he had broken a small bone in his foot in the first five minutes of the game but hadn't told anyone. He played on, which hadn't helped, and then scored the winning goal, which probably had helped neither. To thunderous applause, whoops of delight, the flashes of many cameras, and much singing and shouting we were crowned the Summer Sixes Third Division Soccer Champions. We got free beer tokens for the night and a trophy which we tried not to lose or damage (we didn't leave it at the pub, but we did dent it when Pirate Steve dropped it at our after-party back at Nick's). We were popular winners, as were the Chefs, who'd won Division Four – examples of the everyday man (or everyday football player) who, with an attitude to succeed and some amazing support, can overcome details like a lack of skill or fitness to achieve anything. But, of course, once we had achieved that, after a few drinks we wanted more, and Rick tried surreptitiously, but good-naturedly, to swap our trophy with the First Division winners.

After the pub shut, Rick, our designated driver (this year by choice, not by an impending birth), drove his minibus to Nick's house where we could cool down and have a few quiet beers. Nothing of the sort happened – we heated up and had many loud beers along with stories and songs. Then we had a 'back-farting' festival on the lino of Nick's hallway.

The origins of 'back-farting' remain a mystical and, perhaps sensibly, a mythical secret. The origins may have stemmed from Jim's stepbrother doing sit-ups indoors with no shirt on, when he noticed the squelchy sound that could be made with the skin of his back against the lino-covered floor. Another theory tells of a gathering around a campfire on a beach, when Jim asked if there was any linoleum and, to his complete surprise, someone had a roll in the back of their car. He gave a demonstration of 'back-farting' (on lino, on the beach) that was so successful, the entire party around the campfire lifted their tops and joined in, as Jim led them through a rendition of 'Greensleeves'.

Regardless of its origins, or its potential as a reputable form of music, if you're not already a practitioner, 'back-farting' is a bit out of the ordinary. First, it's best if everyone present has no top on, and their shorts (or skirts) pulled down to the crack. In certain social situations this might be awkward and embarrassing, but for us, that night, hot and sweaty, we were already there. Next, everyone lies on their backs on the floor in a line (preferably on a 'lino' floor – wood also works well, but carpet would be a waste of time). It's amazing the range of different notes you can get from quickly raising and lowering a number of differently shaped sticky backs on and off linoleum. The deepest bass-note back-farter should be at one end, then everyone lies in order of pitch until the final back-farter at the other end has the highest note on the scale. This may take some time with shuffling around, comparing pitch and using the opportunity to take in more fluids. It's a bit confronting at first, like auditioning for a band and not wanting to mess it up. But once you relax it becomes easier. Jim said it was like hula-hooping – 'the less you do, the more you get'.

So Jim, who captained us through three seasons of football, led us to win the third division championship and then led us through our journeys into fatherhood, now coached us on back-farting, and he got a very reasonable rendition of 'Tie Me Kangaroo Down, Sport' out of us.

Later, settled, Jim made a speech thanking everyone for their efforts over the year, and years, before. He took us through each game of this last season; who had scored, and who had won Man of the Match. After every game, each player anonymously nominated a fellow player as Man of the Match – someone they thought had played an outstanding game. Jim kept a secret tally so we could award a Player of the Season trophy. Everyone had won Man of the Match on at least one occasion, but Ross scored the most points from his fellow players and he was a very proud man as he collected what is probably now his most prized possession – a splendidly understated sports trophy with a little golden cartoon-like footballer figure kicking the air. Ross also received a prize, and he was equally pleased with his op-shop vintage coasters and placemats with scenes of the British countryside on them.

Other deserved performances were also rewarded: Chad, who was runner-up for Player of the Season received a skate mag and a rock from Jim's grandad's garden in Ireland; and Nick got skate mags for 'most improved player'.

Then more celebrating – the rum and the vodka appeared – and Jim got the dizzies, and was under the kitchen table even before the tequila came out. We had a big night.

Not highlights by any means, but things that we can now piece together from the night include: watching the DVD highlights reel from season one (probably more than once); moving a very heavy old bath from one end of the garden to the other for Nick; and an interpretive dance competition under the moonlight where you were given a word like 'special' and had to dance an interpretation of that word with only a 3x3 metre piece of blue tarpaulin as a prop.

Nick and Sally had only just moved into this house – the housewarming party was in a few weeks time – but they had graciously made it available to us for the night. Chad, Ben, Nick, Ross and I slept for a few hours on couches or blow-up mattresses (we couldn't tell the difference). Rick was curled up on a towel near the door. Yari somehow ended up in a double bed on his own all night and Pirate Steve was on the picnic table outside. Also outside was Jim, who had crawled from under the kitchen table with his broken foot, down the laundry ramp and found a spot on the lawn next to the veggie patch. Someone covered him with a tablecloth early in the morning so he wouldn't get a chill.

Next morning we woke and squinted around while trying to separate our tongues from the roofs of our mouths. Things looked very different from the way they looked the night before. The huge cast-iron bath we had moved from one side of the garden to the other had left some destruction in its wake. Obstacles that seemed difficult to step over at the end of the night had now miraculously shrunk, or disappeared. And it felt as if we had done five hundred sit-ups with no shirt on.

We needed to go out for a victory breakfast. We chose a restaurant close by where one of the players of the Chefs football team worked. On the specials board he had listed 'Victory Breakfast': so good – although blood pudding certainly must have come across a bit strong after a big night for a vegan like Rick. Afterwards, with glazy eyes and fuzzy heads we said goodbye to each other and dragged our sorry selves home to take on our fatherly duties for the day. Duties that, today especially, might include a little extra because we'd been out all night.

And now the real adventure begins. We don't have babies anymore, we have toddlers who walk and have started to talk. We have little people we need to teach things to. We have important decisions to make, developments to nurture, curiosity to encourage and creativity to cultivate. We have also willingly entered into a never-ending, ever-evolving pact, or contract, with our partners about every single aspect of how to raise a child, from a baby to a young adult.

As a group of blokes, getting together now is usually very different – we still play football together for ten to twelve weeks a year, but we also meet over at the park, or at the beach or on the swings, at the weekends. It's difficult, though, to talk deeply in these situations, so we have recently formed a kind of men's group to ensure we still get together regularly and discuss how we're going. It's training, but of a different type.

I sent an email to the Trombone dads:

> As beautifully happy as I am with my family life – my home is filled with gentle energy, love and oestrogen – something is missing: I need some ball-tearing testosterone time! So, on the last Friday of every month, you are welcome round to my place for sci-fi action films, sport, drinking, smoking, general tool talk and matey chat/support ('what's said in the room stays in the room'), games and strippers (not really, no strippers). I don't think this is turning away from any of my responsibilities and I'm sure it will make me a better partner, father and friend – what do you reckon?

I also added, tongue-in-cheek:

> In order to sound more important and worthwhile to our partners when asking for leave passes, I'm calling this regular piss-up 'Men Understanding Fatherhood' … or MUF. Of course, getting home is a prob, perhaps car share with a DD, share taxis or cycle? I'm not thinking too late or raucous a night, I do have permission but I also have a baby upstairs and Mette says I have to be able the next day. She also says not too many men, but I told her 'I wear the trousers in my house and I'll do what I like when I like!' So, sorry, only two or three at a time – and we have to be really really quiet (not really really).

As the only one without kids, Nick was excluded from this group and wondered what happened at MUF nights. Did we get all primal and start howling at the moon? Or was it more like an AA session? Did we cry? Did we hug each other? Or was it just a lot of beer drinking, back slapping and pocket pissing?

We meet on the last Friday of every month in my backyard. We sit outside my shed around a camp fire – with a wheelbarrow full of ice not far away – to share stories and discuss the issues we each face as new fathers – often the same issues. It's an opportunity to talk and listen; to receive and offer advice; and to identify and empathise with other men.

Initially or partners thought this was merely an excuse to get together for a few beers. Well, it is, but it's so much more than that, too. Ross' wife once mentioned to his aunt that he was going out that Friday night for MUF – she looked horrified. Ross listened as his wife explained, and his aunt said, 'That's exactly what my husband needed. Good on you!'

We have a lot of fun, talk like men and giggle like boys. But we keep on track, discussing our experiences of fatherhood, and I know that the sharing makes us stronger.

I know the other fathers, like me, marvel at the fact that our new baby sons and daughters implicitly understand the most important things in life: simple things, like love and happiness. As new fathers, we all agree that the sound of a child laughing is the most beautiful sound ever. And even a child crying at night is something to be grateful for – their presence. The experience of belonging, learning and doing well as a new father has to make you proud, secure and optimistic for the future, and it makes you live in the 'now' every moment of every day.

It's fair to say we were content as men before season one. We were each happy and content with most aspects of our lives before we met and any of this happened. Now it's fair to say that we are more content than before and importantly, more 'complete'. Looking back on that last season and seeing us become champions is seeing us all as 'winners'. Of course, we were all doing well in the game of life before any of this began; we were all safe, healthy, and in happy relationships. We enhanced that when we met each other and had fun getting to know one another during season one. Then that went to another level in season two when we became fathers together as Fertile FC. Now we were Bangalow Summer-Sixes Third Division champions and had a trophy with our name on it to prove it. And although it was great to win the final, any of us would give it away without a thought for the prize we each now value most – our new baby sons and daughters born during our footballing journey into fatherhood.

EXTRA TIME

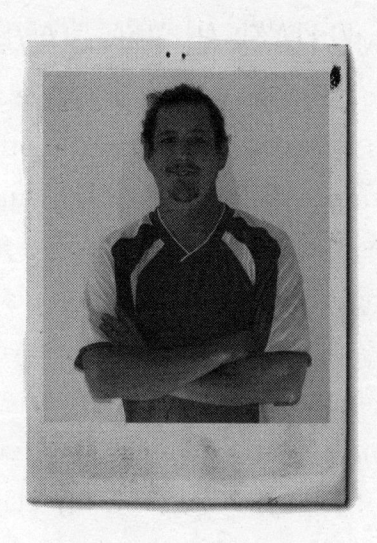

NICK'S STORY

Nicknamed Bootsy because of his unique, old-fashioned football boots, Nick is a left-footed defender, or winger, and loves to go forward on attack. The mix of old boots, mismatched socks and new boardies presents quite a distinctive appearance on the field, and gives the impression that he's not that experienced in the finer points of the game. He was the instigator of the team song and host of the end-of-season champion's party. He's not afraid to have a pop at the opposition's goal if it's in his sights or to hold his ground to protect his own.

OF THE BLOKES WHO PLAYED ALL THREE SEASONS OF SIX-A-SIDE

soccer, I was the only one who didn't have a baby. I'd like to say that's because I'm younger than the other guys and in a recent relationship, but I'm not – I must just be a bit slow. It took me seventeen years to propose to my partner, Sally, and when I rang her father to ask for his daughter's hand in marriage, he replied, 'Well, I think you've done your apprenticeship, mate.'

The first time I met Sally was at a school swimming carnival. One of her sisters was in my class and Sally was a grade below us. I remember clearly the moment when her sister introduced us. Everything went quiet, the screaming crowds blurred into the background, Sally walked slowly towards us shaking the chlorinated water from her long blond hair, our eyes met and that was it. She trotted off and I was in love.

That was two decades ago and we've been together ever since, travelling then working and saving together towards buying our own house. A couple of years ago, we finally managed to gather a deposit for an old house about half an hour from the beach (as close to the beach as we could afford). I proposed to Sally on the night we opened the front door to our new home for the first time.

Thinking back, I suppose it was only a matter of time. Sally and I started talking about having kids years earlier, but it was always based in the distant future when we were grown up. For a long time I was blissfully unaware that I was in fact becoming a grown up. The first inkling of the demise of my own youth came halfway through our travels in Europe. I had long hair back then and was sitting in a bar in France when a couple of young lads sparked up a conversation. After a bit of chit-chat, out of nowhere one of them commented, 'You've got an awesome mullet, man.' Not long after that rude awakening I paid a backpacker (who was carrying hairdressing scissors with her) ten euros to cut it short. Gradually, I started to develop a healthy disregard for Gen Y. Teenagers stopped talking to me, and when they eventually stopped acknowledging my existence all together I came to the shocking realisation that I was a grown up.

When we moved from the Gold Coast, we started spending time with Sarah, an old friend from college who was now living in Mullumbimby. One weekend while camping with a bunch of mates by the beach, Sarah told us she had just met a new man called Jim. 'You'll like Jim, he surfs and he lent me a tent.' Jim and I became mates and I was invited to play for the Rusty Trombones FC.

I enjoyed the football that first season, even though I hadn't played much before. Then the new year rolled along and before the second season started I found out all these new mates had all been playing a few extra games in the bedroom and had all scored. All of them, except for me. But I can honestly say that each time I heard another one of the guys from the team had got one past the keeper it felt like a team goal and something to celebrate by running around with your shirt over your head.

As you can imagine, by the third season I was feeling a bit like the odd one out. For two decades Sally and I had only gone through a few packets of condoms. We used the withdrawal method and every now and then I would find myself wondering whether I was playing with a loaded gun. I don't know whether the team had got together and resolved they would help me fulfil the new selection criteria, but it was around this time they started encouraging me to have a few runs up front during the games. All of a sudden there was a collective and dubious interest to see if I could score a goal. Some nights, during our warm-up kick-around, if I scored a goal they'd all look at me funny and make little comments like, 'Tonight might be the night, mate, hey, hey.'

Even though they call me 'Bootsy' there's nothing magical about my boots or my left foot, but with all the team backing me it was only a matter of time before the magical moment of getting one past the keeper arrived. The ball was traveling up the left side of the field and I was there waiting in my newly appointed position of 'Stand there and wait till we get it past every defender then we'll pass it to you', when the ball appeared at my feet. It was just me and the goalkeeper. I dummied left, I dummied right and then blasted it. The ball came rocketing off my right foot and flew straight into the keeper's nose. The ball dropped to the ground, the keeper dropped to the ground, nose bloodied, and the goal was wide open. I couldn't miss.

News travels pretty fast around Byron Bay, especially through the Trombettes. That night when I got home I discovered Sally at the front door wearing a sly grin and a twinkle in her eye. 'So, I heard you scored tonight, baby' – nudge, nudge, wink, wink. Bada bing bada bang … GOOOOOOOOOOOOOOOOAL!

After all the seasons of me playing football and Sally coming to watch me play, she is now occasionally still seen sitting by the sideline. But now it's with what could easily be mistaken as a soccer ball under her dress. After seventeen years of practising together (and I'm not just talking about soccer), I finally got one past the keeper. I'm still not sure if it had anything to do with the football team, but they do say fertility is catching and maybe in my case it was a long incubation period. Sally wrote the news in the sand while we were walking along the beach, but in my heart I already knew she was pregnant. In fact, I even remember the stroke – I haven't scored many goals in my life and I can remember them all, but I'll save you the details.

On the beach Sally picked up a stick and told me to turn around. I knew she was writing in the sand and I also knew what she was writing. 'Don't look!' she yelled, but I couldn't help myself. I turned around and saw what I already knew was written there. Sally was so happy to tell me but really pissed off that I turned around too soon. She punched my arm, started to cry then hugged me. It took a while for the news to settle in but I was ready and I was stoked. I was also pretty happy that my little swim team had the goods to get across the line.

The Northern Rivers region has a great community vibe, and as well as the football team, there's plenty of other support groups. Even the plumber, a big bloke from Lismore, gave me some advice the other day. The first time he turned up to fix our gas stove he was acting really blokey. 'You should be able to fix this one on your own now, shouldn't ya?' he said to his apprentice, turning back to tell me that he was the boss but he'd just come back to work after taking time off to help the wife out with the new kid. That was about it for conversation that day. A week or so later, though, when he came back with a replacement part, Sally answered the door as she was leaving for work. I came out to the kitchen and he had this goofy smile on his face. 'Mate, you didn't tell me you are having a little baby! You old devil you.' I thought he was going give me a big cuddle. As he was leaving that day, he told me all about how his little boy had been born early and was tiny when he came out: 'But not anymore, you should see him now.' Even the apprentice told me that his mate's missus had the biggest recorded baby born in Lismore hospital.

'You're going to be the most informed father-to-be ever, Nick,' Neil said the other day. Being the last in the team, I've heard about caesareans, cervical lips wrapped over heads, twisted shoulders and screaming babies. With the team I've debated the pros and cons of vaccination and shared tips on clearing up nipple infections. I've listened to them bragging about who's got the best swaddling technique, reminiscing over trusty old cots passed down through the family, mourning the ones that were thrown out and missed forever, and also revealing the ancient secrets of the Indian baby-soothing technique (step forward one, two, three, lunge down, step back two, three, lunge down).

Ross pulled Sally and me up after a recent game, sausage sanga in hand. He said sincerely, 'Nick and Sal, make sure you make the most of these times together because it's all going to change soon. So just make sure, okay?' Everyone in the team told me that I'd have no time after the baby arrives, and they're probably right, but maybe I'll just gain the magical power they now have, and restructure my business with one hand while wiping baby sick up with the other. Rick usually has a good yarn, and being a pro in the baby-making department he could have been telling all the lads what to expect, but like an old sage he just stood back and proclaimed, 'Every birth is different, boys.'

I can honestly say that I'm ready to have this baby. I know I have the easy job – but it's not as easy as it used to be when the prospective father got to sit in the waiting room with a bottle of Scotch and a cigar. But listening to all the different experiences while playing for Fertile FC has taught me some valuable lessons. As I prepare for the most important game I've ever played, the three golden rules I have learned through three seasons of six-a-side football while becoming a budding father are: teamwork, preparation and support.

First, teamwork: make sure you and your partner are both on the same side at all times. Play well together and stay united, even when you are exhausted and may be feeling unappreciated. After a football game, a wise man once said, 'Look after your relationship, and the baby will then be looked after well.' Check in with each other regularly. Don't just let one day become the next and don't spend all your time together talking about mundane duties and responsibilities.

Preparation is the second skill to master: know what to expect, but then expect the unexpected. Do everything you can beforehand to make your lives as ready as possible. Travel, visit friends for dinner, go and see lots of movies, fix that old washer on the kitchen sink; apparently what everybody says is true – you won't have much free time after the baby arrives. All the new fathers I've spoken to also experienced another phenomenon, and Sally and I have too. It's commonly known as 'nesting', but I refer to it by its other name – 'renovating'. It starts as a strong and undeniable urge to visit Bunnings and ends up consuming every spare weekend for the last two trimesters of pregnancy.

And finally, support: during the pregnancy, remember that only the best fish and chips in town will do. Serve it up with one hand while adjusting the pillow behind her head with the other, as she reclines sleepily on the couch for two months. And once the baby is home, there will be some new jobs especially for you. You will be the water bringer, shopping getter, cloth fetcher, laundry taker-outerer and folder-upperer. This position is seven days a week with no paid overtime. And best to do all this with a big smile (see point one: teamwork).

Performance anxiety is inevitable and so are the little tears that appear out of nowhere. They may arise for all kinds of reasons and are impossible to pinpoint. So don't be too concerned if she starts sobbing when you comment that the tray of mangoes you just bought are a bit overripe this time. It will pass (don't forget point two: support).

There are also some great times to be had. Sally and I, like all the other couples in the team, really enjoyed reading the books that outline the development of the foetus. After each week's chapter, Sally and I would come up with a new name for our little lentil, who slowly progressed from a chickpea to a jalapeño, banana, etc. Eventually, Sally drew the line at pumpkin, preferring instead 'apple head'.

Ultimately, it's all about the little one who is coming into the world for the first time. Neil said to me once, 'Be prepared to fall in love like you never have before.' Contemplating the idea of my own child coming into the world has me hoping above all that every new father will have enough love to give to every new child who arrives.

ADDED TIME IN EXTRA TIME

Nick and Sally now have a healthy baby boy, Reuben.

Suggested Further Reading

Man with a Pram by Jon Farry and Stephen Mitchell
These people know what they're talking about and it shows. It has an index so you can look things up and it's laid out in order, but it's not like you have to start at the beginning. You can flick through and find interesting stuff in sidebars and boxes. It has pictures and trivia, lots of stats and helpful hints, all told with wisdom and a dash of wit. It's the next book to read now you've finished this one – while she reads *Up the Duff*. – **Neil**

I was given *Man with a Pram* when Sally and I were still preparing to have our little racing-car driver, and although it doesn't actually give any tips on how to pimp my pram, it was really helpful when it came to those more important aspects of having a baby, from conception to birth. I didn't need any help with the first bit, that's for sure, but the closer it got to D-Day the more Sally could be heard commenting, 'He's reading that book again.' There's one chapter that starts with something like, 'If you are just thinking about this part of the birth at this stage in your partner's pregnancy, panic now!' I remained calm and collected, however, and read the chapter really quickly before Sally found out. Neil read a bit of it the other day and said that it was the book we all needed when we were pregnant for the first time. It's written by a bloke who teaches writing and a male nurse, who became fathers and discovered, like we did over beers at the pub, that there aren't many books out there for blokes about how to have babies written by blokes who have just had babies. They do a great job with this book – it gives you a good idea about how it all works and what you're in for as an expectant father. It has heaps of helpful tips to support your pregnant missus and, most of all, it helps you relax and enjoy the best moment of your life. – **Nick**

The Dad Factor by Richard Fletcher

Richard is the leader of the Fathers and Families Research Program at the University of Newcastle and has been doing heaps of research and writing on family matters from the Newcastle University Family Action Centre for many years now.

In his book *The Dad Factor*, Richard discusses bonding, new brain research, the fear-based climate surrounding children's active play and the loss of respect for fatherhood. He concludes that fathering is not the same as mothering; there are important differences in the way we bond with our children that are equally important to their future wellbeing. Richard does all this in a very easy and accessible way with lots of stories and examples.

As a new dad, I found this book really interesting and would highly recommend it to anyone who likes some science, theory and research behind their reading. The generation of fathers before us didn't have access to any of this information when they fathered us. We can be so much better educated and prepared by sharing our stories with other fathers and having a background of supportive evidence. – **Neil**

***From Here to Paternity* by *Sydney Morning Herald* journalist Sacha Molitorisz**

This was the only book I found that was a real story from a real man about how he felt as he went through the process of childbirth. Ross passed it on to me and I enjoyed it and got a lot out of it. It's told in a lighthearted way, but it is only one man's story, and if you don't relate to his life, relationship and frame of mind, then it may not be so interesting. It's a diary-like account of his experience, interspersed with some history and facts, and for that alone, it's definitely worth a read. **– Neil**

Bella found this book for me and thought it would be one that I might actually read. I did, and really enjoyed it. The author has researched many different aspects of the pregnancy experience, so it was a bit like having a study pal to cheat from. The information was useful and varied. He's a good writer and it was an easy read, so I passed it on to mates. **– Ross**

***Up the Duff: The Real Guide to Pregnancy* by Kaz Cooke**

A humorous book, which makes it a good read, and very Australian. But like most pregnancy books out there, it's written by a woman for womankind. I didn't relate to the diary part of it at all, but the way Kaz gives facts, advice and useful information – with humour – makes it easily digestible for a bloke. Recommend it to your partner and have a read if you find it on her bedside table. **– Neil**

***What's Inside Your Tummy, Mummy?* by Abby Cocovini**
A great book to show kids what is happening to their mum. Each week of the pregnancy is described with a scale picture of something to denote the size of the baby (such as a watermelon at the end of the pregnancy). It helps to bring existing kids into the process and to alleviate any issues of sibling jealousy. – **Jim**

***Spiritual Midwifery* by Ina May Gaskin**
This book was quite an eye-opener for me. It starts off with three hundred people travelling the USA in old school buses, stopping for 'caravan births' when women went into labour. It showed us, a little extremely, how some people outside mainstream society give birth in a calm, conscious way with the full safety of medical training and supervision. Written by midwives from the Farm community in Tennessee, it apparently became a classic on the natural birthing scene when it was first published in 1975. In particular, I liked the birth stories, which were very detailed and from both parents' perspectives, and often so outrageous (breech babies, babies in the back of vans in freezing winters, etc.) it made our impending birth seem very tame and easy. – **Yari**

***New Active Birth* by Janet Balaskas**
This is not the kind of book I'd pick up in a bookshop, but it sure made both our kids' births that much easier. It encourages the woman in labour to walk around, squat, lie down and move in any way she wants during labour. I mean, lying on your back

can't be the best way to push a baby out, it defies gravity! It's full of common sense and not too 'out there' (unlike *Spiritual Midwifery*). – **Yari**

Your Pregnancy Week by Week by Professor Lesley Regan

Big and shiny with lots of factual information, statistics and impressive colour photographs, all with full references to current international medical knowledge – makes you go 'wow'. But then the more you read, the more frightened you become about this enormous thing you're about to go through. Good to buy for your partner if you want to show you care. We read it together – the corresponding chapter each week of our pregnancy – and it did bring us closer and ensured that she knew that I knew what she wanted me to know. – **Neil**

Baby Love by Robin Barker

Expert Australian advice for the first twelve months of a baby's life. We used this book a lot in the first days and weeks after bringing our new baby home. You can look things up in the index and there are sections for the first days, the first weeks, etc. Mostly, reading it allowed me to relax and see that there's a wide range of 'normal'. It was a source of good advice and meant we didn't always have to drive out to the doctor or midwife or local nurse to ask another stupid question. It also contains lots of advice on baby nutrition (including recipes), allergies, safe sleeping, breastfeeding, immunisation and all that stuff that you know nothing about until you're in the middle of it. – **Neil**

The Magical Child by Joseph Chilton Pearce

This recommendation comes with a warning – this book puts very complex ideas forward in a way that's often difficult to understand. When Sarah told me that I should read it because it resonated with her parenting style, I dropped everything to read it, as any dutiful husband would. It took me a while (about fifty pages) to fully grasp what the author was talking about – he has quite an abstract and esoteric style. The basic idea is that everything we are currently doing in the modern world regarding baby rearing – from the very moment the baby comes into the world and is hit with bright fluorescent lights – is in stark contrast to what the infant actually wants and needs. The baby wants to stay with its mother until it knows it is safe from harm – potentially at least a year. This concept resonated so deeply with me that I felt I needed to recommend it to anyone considering having a baby, but if you can find the concise edition of the *Magical Child* go for that first. – Jim

Vaccination Roulette: Experiences, Risks and Alternatives **produced by the Australian Vaccination Network**

This book is produced by the Australian Vaccination Network (a group obviously against vaccination), so I must advise that it is slightly biased, in my opinion, towards anti-vaccination. It is also full of stats and jargon that is not really needed. But I do recommend this book to anyone considering vaccinating their child. The stories of people who have experienced the side effects of a vaccine straight after having it are definitely worth reading. Some of the stories are truly quite disturbing. – **Jim**

The Vaccination Book **by Robert Sears**
With publicity surrounding the possible health risks posed by childhood immunisation, parents are no longer simply following doctors' orders and automatically having their children vaccinated; instead, they are asking questions. The problem is the search for answers only leads to conflicting, one-sided information. This book claims that parents finally have one fair, impartial, fact-based resource they can turn to for answers. Dr Bob Sears is neither pro-vaccine nor anti-vaccine and each chapter is devoted to a disease/vaccine and offers comprehensive detailed information. – **Neil**

WEBSITES

Calmbirth (childbirth preparation program)
www.calmbirth.com.au

Bonnie Babes Foundation (dealing with birth loss)
www.bbf.org.au

THANKS

Thanks to all of us, from each of us in the team, for being so honest and open about our experiences. We've all learned heaps and sharing our stories makes us better fathers and partners.

Big thanks to all the partners of the men in the team, for allowing us to be so honest and open about our experiences – the mothers of future Australian footballers: Sarah, Nella, Bella, Christina, Mette and Sally.

To all the doctors, midwives and staff who help parents give birth.

The forgotten Rusty Trombones from season one: Tom and Hamish.

The forgotten Fertile from season two: Heinz.

Scott Kruegar, Paul Hanigan and Glen Hanigan and their friends and family for organising the Bangalow Summer Sixes. The other teams and everyone who came and cut up oranges, played the trombone, filmed us or watched us play football.

Also thanks to Alan Close, the Northern Rivers Writers' Centre and the Byron Bay Writers' Festival where the idea for this book was first pitched. Terry Bleakley and Bleak Films. Bernadette Foley, Jacquie Brown, Kate Stevens and everyone else at Hachette Australia.

THE FERTILE FC BLOG

This book covers just the beginning of our journeys into fatherhood. Since having children we realise that you have to live in the 'now', and that the challenges, joys, duties and surprises change daily. Through our fathers' group we are lucky enough to have conversations with other men at least monthly. We wanted to share some of the stories that come up at these meetings with a wider audience to further contribute to the open and honest discussions men are having with each other about their situations and feelings, particularly in relation to their partners and children.

For our blog, we take it in turns to write something each week. Something that is relevant to us as our babies become toddlers, something important to us in our everyday lives, and usually an ordinary topic told with a father's insight and a man's humour. We hope this becomes a forum for other fathers to read and contribute to; to join with us as we become more comfortable and confident being present and engaging at every stage of our child's development, from pregnancy through to baby, toddler and forward into the future.

Our blogsite also has heaps of interesting links to other useful sites.

blog: www.fertile.com

One Got Past the Keeper
www.facebook.com/fertilefc

@fertilefc

ABOUT THE FATHERHOOD PROJECT

We always wanted to give a percentage of any money earned from this book to a worthy cause. Our favourite not-for-profit organisations are all born in the Northern Rivers area where we live and all involve strengthening families. We highly commend the work of Uncle – a community-based mentoring and activities program for local boys without active fathers (www.uncle.org.au); Pathways to Manhood – a contemporary rites of passage program for boys and girls (www.pathwaysfoundation.com.au); and our chosen beneficiary, with which this book is most closely aligned, the Fatherhood Project (www.fatherhood.net.au).

The Fatherhood Project is a not-for-profit organisation that supports fathers to be actively and positively engaged in their children's lives. Its aim is to improve the health and wellbeing of children, families and communities. The Fatherhood Project develops and delivers specialised education, support and mentoring programs for fathers, including expectant fathers, young fathers (aged sixteen to twenty-five), long-distance dads (who are working away from home) and indigenous fathers.

It was established in the Northern Rivers area in 2003 and has quickly become known nationwide through the Fatherhood Festival. It has delivered programs for fathers from the Pilbara mines in Western Australia and Melbourne's City of Casey to Queensland's Gold Coast, all with one theme – supporting and educating fathers in their most important role.

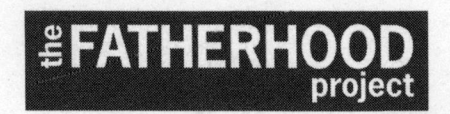

the FATHERHOOD project   www.fatherhood.net.au